D1713433

Ticlopidine, Platelets and Vascular Disease

Ticlopidine Hydrochloride

5-(2-chlorophenyl)methyl]-4,5,6,7-tetrahydrothieno [3,2-c] pyridine hydrochloride.

William K. Hass   J. Donald Easton
Editors

Ticlopidine, Platelets and Vascular Disease

With 20 Illustrations

Springer-Verlag
New York Berlin Heidelberg London Paris
Tokyo Hong Kong Barcelona Budapest

William K. Hass, MD
Department of Neurology
New York University School of Medicine
New York, NY 10016
USA

J. Donald Easton, MD
Department of Neurology
Brown University Medical Center
Providence, RI 02903
USA

Library of Congress Cataloging-in-Publication Data
Ticlopidine, platelets and vascular disease / William K. Hass,
   J. Donald Easton, editors.
      p.   cm.
   Includes bibliographical references and index.
   ISBN 0-387-94009-X. — ISBN 3-540-94009-X
   1. Ticlopidine—Testing.   2. Blood-platelets—Aggregation.
   3. Cerebrovascular disease—Chemotherapy.   4. Myocardial infarction—
Chemotherapy. I. Hass, William K., 1929– .   II. Easton, J. Donald.
      [DNLM: 1. Blood Platelets—physiology.   2. Ticlopidine—
therapeutic use.   3. Vascular Diseases—drug therapy.   WG 500 T557
1993]
   RM666.T55T53   1993
   616.1061—dc20
   DNLM/DLC
   for Library of Congress   92–48386

Printed on acid-free paper.

© 1993 Springer-Verlag New York Inc.

Production coordinated by Chernow Editorial Services, Inc. and managed by
   Henry Krell; manufacturing supervised by Jacqui Ashri.
Typeset by Typographic Specialties, Bozeman, MT.
Printed and bound by Edwards Brothers, Inc., Ann Arbor, MI.
Printed in the United States of America.

9 8 7 6 5 4 3 2 1

ISBN 0-387-94009-X Springer-Verlag New York Berlin Heidelberg
ISBN 3-540-94009-X Springer-Verlag Berlin Heidelberg New York

Preface

Blood platelets lack a nucleus. As a result their life span is short and they cannot reproduce themselves. Platelets share these qualities with the red blood cell. Platelets and red blood cells, nevertheless, serve vital roles in the body. One major function of the platelet is its capacity to aggregate and thereby initiate intravascular coagulation which often underlies such major diseases as myocardial infarction, cerebral infarction, and pulmonary embolism. For this reason in recent years, medical attention has been directed to drugs that inhibit platelet aggregation.

Aspirin was the first drug to be proven effective in this area. Since then other drugs that share aspirin's fundamental biochemical action, inhibition of platelet cyclooxygenase, have also been studied. Very recently, ticlopidine, the first of what promises to be a new class of drugs inhibiting platelet aggregation and coagulation via an entirely different biochemical mechanism, has been extensively studied and clinically shown to be as effective or more effective than aspirin in the prevention of ischemic cardiovascular and cerebrovascular disease.

The medical world knows and understands aspirin well. It has been widely available to physicians and patients for almost a century. Ticlopidine, on the other hand, is novel and has not been the subject of a formal and rigorous textbook review. Increasingly widespread use of ticlopidine throughout the world now requires such an effort. Having been assured of the cooperation of the authors of the individual chapters, all of whom enjoy international reputations for their expertise in their assigned areas of review, the editors undertook this effort fully aware that books so designed are not read like novels. Most physicians will, no doubt, approach this book with specific questions in mind and address themselves largely to one or two chapters of immediate interest. This makes some repetition from chapter to chapter necessary. Efforts have been made, however, to minimize repetition for those who would like to peruse this volume in depth.

The book is, therefore, dedicated to a wide spectrum of physicians considering treatment of patients with ticlopidine, perhaps for the first time, who will find herein an in-depth presentation of information necessary for confident medical care.

William K. Hass, M.D.
J. Donald Easton, M.D.

Contents

Contributors

Francesco Balsano, MD, Università degli Studi di Roma "La Sapienza," Istituto di I Clinica Medica, 00161 Rome, Italy.

John Bruno, PH.D, Consultant in Thrombosis and Atherosclerosis Research, Palo Alto, CA 94304, USA.

J. Donald Easton, MD, Professor, Department of Neurology, Brown University, Providence, RI 02903, USA.

Michael Gent, Professor, McMaster University and the Hamilton Civic Hospitals Research Centre, Hamilton, Ontario L8V 1C3, Canada.

Laurence A. Harker, MD, Professor, Division of Hematology and Oncology, Emory University School of Medicine, Atlanta, GA 30322, USA.

William K. Hass, MD, Professor, Department of Neurology, New York University Medical Center, New York, NY 10016, USA.

Lars Janzon, MD, Department of Community Health Sciences, Lund University, Malmö General Hospital, Malmö, Sweden.

Basil A. Molony, MD, Internist, Clinical Trialist, Los Altos, CA 94024, USA.

Edouard Panak, Sanofi Pharma, 32-34 Rue Marbeuf 7500, 75008 Paris, France.

William Pryse-Phillips, MD, Professor, Department of Medicine, Division of Neurology, St. Johns, Newfoundland A1B 3V6, Canada.

Philip Teitelbaum, PH.D, Head, Department of Drug Metabolism, Syntex Discovery Research, Palo Alto, CA 94304, USA.

Monique Verry, PH.D, Sanofi Pharma, 32-34 Rue Marbeuf 7500, 75008 Paris, France.

Francesco Violi, MD, Università degli Studi di Roma, "La Sapienza," Istituto di I Clinica Medica, 00161 Rome, Italy.

1
Changing Concepts of the Pathophysiology of Cerebral and Myocardial Infarction

WILLIAM K. HASS and J. DONALD EASTON

Introduction

In this volume we shall review the current status of antiplatelet therapy for vascular occlusive disease. Specific attention will be paid to the first of a new class of antiplatelet agents, ticlopidine hydrochloride. Our observations will be timebound and therefore imperfect. Imperfection, however, has its virtues. In 1991 Ordinas[1] noted that a fully suppressive antiplatelet agent would be so effective, so perfect, that the adverse effect of severe bleeding would be the likely result of its administration. A perfect drug, in fact, is more likely to be classified as a poison than as a proper and safe medication.

In contrast to such a fully suppressive agent, ticlopidine at physiologic doses does not completely inhibit platelet activity. In humans on a relatively small daily dose of 375 mg, there is only a 60–70% diminution of ADP-induced platelet aggregation, only a moderate increase in template bleeding time, and incomplete (therefore imperfect) protection against A–V shunt occlusion[2] (Figure 1.1).

Progressing further on the trail of imperfection, we shall present in detail three recently reported major clinical trials[3–5] showing that ticlopidine: 1) is more effective than a placebo in the prevention of recurrent stroke, myocardial infarction, and vascular death in patients who suffered a completed stroke (Canadian American Ticlopidine Study—CATS); 2) is significantly more effective than aspirin for reducing the risk of stroke after transient ischemic attacks, amaurosis fugax, and minor stroke (Ticlopidine Aspirin Stroke Study—TASS); and 3) is strikingly effective in reducing the risk of fatal and nonfatal myocardial infarction in patients with unstable angina (STAI).

In none of the cited studies, however, does risk reduction even approach perfection, i.e., 100% risk reduction. Given the incomplete suppression of platelet aggregation by ticlopidine at physiologic doses and the less-than-total reduction in stroke risk, it is not surprising that the usefulness of ticlopidine in contrast to aspirin in the prevention of stroke or myocardial infarction has excited commentary from medical editorialists.[6,7] Thus FitzGerald has asked, "Is ticlopidine merely a 'more expensive aspirin' for use in unstable angina?" He has also correctly pointed out that adverse drug effects were relatively uncommon with

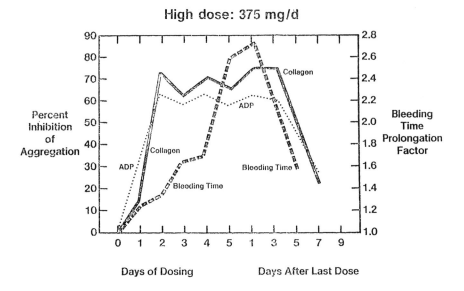

FIGURE 1.1. Patterns of aggregation inhibition in percent or bleeding time prolongation as a time multiple of normal during a ticlopidine onset-offset study in humans. (Courtesy of Dr. David Ellis.)

both ticlopidine and aspirin. Warlow's critique in the *Journal of Neurology, Neurosurgery, Psychiatry* was limited to the problem of stroke prevention. He was bothered by the primary employment of efficacy analysis in the CATS, pointing out that efficacy studies provide the most optimistic estimate of treatment effect. Thus, in the CATS findings risk reduction (ticlopidine vs. placebo of the composite endpoint—stroke, myocardial infarction, vascular death) was 23.3%, a statistically significant level with, however, a wide confidence interval of 1.0–40.5%. The wide confidence level, the fact that 12% of patients stopped taking ticlopidine because of side effects, and the probable cost of the drug in comparison to over-the-counter aspirin led Warlow to opt for aspirin. The Antiplatelet Trialists Collaboration[8] found aspirin to have a mean composite vascular endpoint risk reduction when compared to placebo of 25% with narrow confidence intervals as evaluated by the technique of meta-analysis, which will be examined in detail in a later chapter.

    Thus, forcing a choice between ticlopidine and aspirin is fast becoming a kind of parlor game having little bearing on the real problem—the specific patient with specific risks of an arterial occlusive event. Aspirin, like ticlopidine, is significantly and *also* incompletely effective. It, too, is imperfect. In head-on comparisons for reducing risk of stroke, ticlopidine wins, but not by an overwhelming margin. In short, both drugs are imperfect but both will serve. Both

TABLE 1.1. Blindly adjudicated pathophysiological mechanisms for stroke first events seen in TASS in patients assigned to ticlopidine or aspirin treatment.

Characterization of stroke mechanism	Ticlopidine group (N=1529)	Aspirin group (N=1540)
Type		
Atherothrombotic	104	132
Hemorrhagic infarction	3	4
Cardioembolic	5	6
Lacunar infarction	10	17
Retinal infarction	7	11
Intracerebral hemorrhage	7	7
Uncertain	36	35

exhibit the virtues of imperfection. They will both be extensively discussed in this volume.

The Cerebral Infarction Problem

Our pathophysiological concept of that most-common variety of stroke, athero-thrombotic brain infarction, has also been imperfect (Table 1.1). This concept's history proves, on close examination, to be a struggle of medical-scientific faith against an ever-changing background of medical theory and medical fact. There-fore, we shall record the history of that struggle and survey its current status.

Early in the 20th century, autopsy studies and J. Ramsay Hunt's[8] observation that a lost carotid arterial pulse in patients presenting with "cerebral intermittent claudication," characterized by contralateral episodes of weakness and eventual completed stroke in that arterial territory, strongly suggested that occlusive disease, probably thrombotic, was the basis for ischemic stroke. This conception has informed most of the subsequent efforts to prevent intraarterial occlusion, initially with anticoagulant and more recently with antiplatelet therapy. It has also become the basis for establishing the significance of carotid endarterectomy for stroke prevention in patients having 70–99% stenosis of a carotid artery and having symptoms of cerebral dysfunction related to that artery during the previous 3 months.[10,11]

Therefore, it will come as a surprise, particularly to physicians and surgeons who began to practice medicine after 1970, that *a point-for-point relationship* between arterial stenosis or occlusion to an infarct in the territory of that artery has only been proven to be reasonably valid in the past few years, i.e., 1987–1991. Only 40 years ago Hicks and Warren of the Harvard Medical School challenged the concept that infarcts of the brain were usually caused by thrombosis, describing this item of apparent scientific fact as one of the "most common misconceptions" still widely taught.[12]

Hicks and Warren described 100 autopsied cases from the New England Deaconess Hospital and the Peter Bent Brigham Hospital in Boston, Massachusetts, performed prior to November 1951, in a paper titled "Infarction of the Brain without Thrombosis." All cases selected were those in which stroke was either the principal cause of death or one of the primary causes of death. Among the 100 autopsied cases, thrombosis of cerebral vessels accounted completely for the infarct in only 33 cases and only partially in an additional 7 cases. Sixty percent of the patients, therefore, had "no thrombosis, and a total of 67 cases—two-thirds—required some other pathophysiological explanation than the one usually given, namely thrombosis." The authors concluded that the major mechanism responsible for non-hemorrhagic stroke was not thrombosis but rather a local change in vascular caliber, such as spasm, vasoparalysis or a result of systemic circulatory failure.

The problem was next taken up by Yates and Hutchinson[13] and summarized in their classic monograph in 1961 emphasizing the role of stenosis of the extracranial cerebral arteries in the causation of cerebral infarction. These authors performed full postmortem examinations on 100 cases of clinically diagnosed cerebral ischemia. Cerebral infarction was found in 35 patients among whom there were 74 separate infarcts, 16 of which were in the cerebellum. According to their findings, "Only 22 of the infarcts and 19 of the cases were associated with significant stenosis or occlusion of the extracranial cerebral arteries."

Thus the authors succinctly addressed the crux of the problem, i.e., failure to find a point-for-point *distal* arterial occlusion-to-infarct relationship in most cases of brain infarction. In contrast, there was the extraordinary frequency in all but 3 of the 35 cases of concurrent significant stenosis or occlusion of extracranial cerebral arteries—a provocative finding that added to the growing excitement about a potential vascular surgical role in stroke prevention and the angiographic definition of these lesions.

Increasingly safe and successful four-vessel angiography as a basis for potential surgical removal of extracranial carotid lesions provided the basis for an extensive study of the relationship during life of extracranial and intracranial occlusive disease in patients with transient minor or completed ischemic strokes.[14] Angiographic studies of more than 4,700 patients with stroke symptoms, enrolled in the Joint Study of Extracranial Arterial Occlusion, verified the findings of Yates and Hutchinson. Still, the question of the precise relationship of proximal stenoses or occlusions to distal intracranial infarct remained unsettled. Complicating the problem was the presence of similar lesions, stenotic or occlusive, in large numbers of patients with no symptoms appropriate to the diseased artery.

Many clues, however, were simultaneously appearing about the relationship between cardiac and extracranial arterial lesions and intracranial infarcts. Angiographers during that period remarked that the angiography was often done days to weeks after onset of transient or persistent strokes in patients. This provided time for clot fragmentation or lysis from known *cardiac* sources.[15] Further, on some rare (largely accidental) occasions, transient monocular blindness was observed by funduscopic examination during an episode.[16,17] Therefore, it became clear during the '60s that artery-to-artery embolism from white, mixed, or red thrombus, adherent to underlying atheromatous lesions at the carotid bifurcation, was a significant mechanism for distal transient ocular or cerebral symptoms and, presumably, for persistent infarction when the friable thrombus did not break up quickly or collateral circulation was inadequate to maintain focal brain tissue viability.

Such elegant demonstrations, however, continued to fail to impress many physicians because major angiographic efforts demonstrated major stenotic lesions in symptomatic patients in only one-third of all right or left carotids examined at their origins, and complete occlusions at these sites in only 8% of all extracranial carotid arteries.[14]

It remained for Fieschi and his colleagues in Rome to catch the bird on the wing only three years ago.[18] This study was published almost 40 years after Hicks and Warren raised their serious doubts. It should also be viewed against the background of the recent American Stroke Data Bank Studies, which *failed* to find the causal mechanism for demonstrated cerebral infarcts in 32% of 1,805 patients.[19,20] Fieschi et al. performed cerebral angiographic studies within 4 hours of stroke onset on patients who had ischemic brain infarcts documented on computed tomogram (CT). In all, 80 patients were studied prospectively; all gave a history of a carotid arterial territory first stroke. Patients over 80 years of age were excluded. A normal internal carotid artery or middle cerebral artery, appropriate to the fresh infarction, were found in less than one-quarter (24%) of patients examined during the acute stage of ischemic stroke. In contrast, 61 patients (76%) showed an *occlusion* in the internal carotid artery, middle cerebral artery, or middle cerebral arterial branch *appropriate* to the demonstrated infarct and the patient's symptoms. Most of these lesions were thought to be embolic. The embolic source was attributed to the heart in 17 patients, to the proximal carotid territory appropriate to the infarction in 30 cases, and to the heart or the proximal carotid territory in 20 patients. Primary distal occlusion was seen in 13 cases in whom no proximal embolic source of thrombus could be identified. Thus, scientific faith was vindicated. Preventive therapy with antiplatelet drugs, already widely employed, was provided with a more secure pathophysiologic base.

However, a stubborn group of ischemic strokes, up to 24% based on the data of Fieschi et al., remain resistant to accurate causal characterization. Migraine and lacunar infarcts account for only some of these; thorough understanding remains incompletely and imperfectly realized.

The Myocardial Infarction Problem

In contrast, cardiologists have come further in assessing the pathophysiology of arterial processes proximate to stable angina, unstable angina, and myocardial infarction than have most neurologists in understanding the arterial processes proximate to TIA, crescendo TIA, and cerebral infarction.

Stable Angina Pectoris

It has been known for many years that a history of classic angina is highly predictive of underlying coronary artery atherosclerosis. Stable angina is usually associated with fixed, obstructive coronary artery atherosclerosis resulting in impaired coronary artery flow. Some patients have an element of superimposed arterial vasospasm that accentuates the ischemia. Under various circumstances (e.g., physical exertion) a mismatch occurs between myocardial oxygen demand and coronary blood flow. Nitroglycerin and other nitrates often relieve the mismatch by a series of effects, i.e., decreasing systemic arterial pressure, decreasing left ventricular volume and diastolic pressure, decreasing ejection time, and vasodilating coronary arteries. Beta-adrenergic and calcium channel blocking agents also have important beneficial effects on the heart for preventing angina. Platelet and fibrin thrombi appear to play little or no role in stable angina. Thus, the process seems to be primarily hemodynamic (flow related) rather than thrombotic.

Pathophysiology of Myocardial Infarction and Unstable Angina

Myocardial infarction with normal coronary arteries is infrequent. Occasionally it occurs with profound systemic hypotension or hypoxia, a striking increase in coronary artery vasomotor tone, embolism from a proximal source, or during exercise with aortic stenosis. Myocardial infarction is usually caused by coronary artery disease. The finding of severe atherosclerosis, with and without thrombosis, has been associated with myocardial infarction for many years. However, it was not until the late 1970s that a number of autopsy and angiographic studies established that intracoronary thrombi were the basis of most acute transmural myocardial infarctions.[21] These were not simply attacks of severe angina that resulted in infarction. Rather, thrombosis regularly occurred. Within another year or two it was learned that spontaneous thrombolysis commonly occurs but is often delayed until the tissue is infarcted. When patients are angiogrammed within 4h of a transmural MI, total occlusion is found in 80–85%. By 12–24h, 65% are occluded and by 2 weeks only 35% remain occluded. Angiography done within 5 minutes may show occlusion in nearly 100%. By the mid-1980s it became clear that intracoronary thrombi were also the basis of unstable angina and most nontransmural myocardial infarctions.[21,22] Thus it seemed atherothrombosis (intracoronary thrombus superimposed on an atherosclerotic plaque) was usually the basis for severe unstable angina, nontransmural, and transmural myocardial infarction. The resulting specific outcome may be a function of total obstruction duration, as well as size and extent of the coronary artery or branch involved, and of the availability of collateral circulation.

Recognition of coronary thrombosis, evolving and resolving prior to, during and after these events, is the basis for exploration of the mechanisms initiating and sustaining the thrombotic event. This is necessary for developing medical and surgical therapies for preventing and treating intracoronary thrombi.

Pathophysiology of Thrombosis and Thrombolysis[23]

Recent studies of patients with acute myocardial infarction have shown a high incidence of atherosclerotic plaque rupture.[23-25] Evidence for plaque rupture comes from angiography (i.e., demonstration of "eccentric stenosis with irregular borders"), angioscopy, and autopsy. Precisely what initiates plaque rupture is unknown. Rupture of an atherosclerotic plaque releases tissue factors into the circulation that induce local platelet aggregation, increase coronary vasomotor tone, and ultimately precipitate coronary thrombosis. Thrombus may be occlusive at the onset of symptoms, with later changes resulting in its becoming subocclusive and slowly being spontaneously lysed or removed by fluid dynamic forces. Local vessel arterial wall-related thrombogenic risk factors at the time of coronary plaque disruption, in association with systemic agonists, may control or moderate thrombus formation, growth, and stabilization on the ruptured plaque, thus inducing the various associated pathologic and clinical syndromes.

At the time of plaque disruption, the presence of only a limited number of thrombogenic risk factors may lead to formation of a small thrombus with subsequent fibrotic organization and slow stepwise plaque growth. Presence of more risk factors may lead to an occlusive but labile thrombus, and so to unstable angina or nontransmural infarction. Focal vasoconstriction, variations in oxygen demand, and the degree of collateral supply also contribute to variable presentations of the acute syndromes.

When the thrombus completely occludes the coronary artery, the result is myocardial infarction. A thrombus that does not completely occlude the artery more commonly causes unstable angina. If the thrombus is small and the coronary artery is large, there may be no clinical sequelae other than growth of the coronary lesion. Although plaque rupture is believed to be a common underlying event in acute myocardial infarction, other mechanisms of luminal reduction in the setting of coronary atherosclerotic lesions may be causative in some patients.

Persistent thrombotic occlusion leads to transmural myocardial infarction in the distribution of the involved coronary artery. The actual size of the necrotic area will depend on the size of the coronary bed affected and the extent of collateral blood flow from adjacent coronary arteries. If the coronary thrombus incompletely occludes the artery, lyses spontaneously or is lysed by therapy, the resultant infarct may only involve the subendocardium of the region supplied by the affected artery.

Specific risk factors at the time of plaque disruption influence the degree of thrombogenicity and therefore the onset of various clinical syndromes. One of these risk factors is shear stress. Platelet deposition and thrombus growth after vascular injury are influenced by the high levels of shear stress that exist in close proximity in the presence of advanced vascular lesions. Platelet deposition escalates substantially with increasing stenosis in the presence of the same vascular injury, indicating shear-rate-induced cell activation. In addition, continuous imaging of the blood–vascular wall interaction indicates that the apex, and not the flow recirculation zone distal to the apex, is the segment of greatest platelet accumulation. These data suggest that severity of acute platelet response to plaque disruption will depend, in part, on the sudden change in degree of stenosis after rupture and on the occurrence of the rupture at the apex of preexisting plaque.

Another risk factor is degree of plaque injury at time of rupture. Exposure of deendothelialized vessel wall to perfusing blood at a high shear rate induces platelet deposition and mural thrombosis. The thrombus may be labile and can be dislodged by the perfusing blood flow. Exposure of collagen to blood produces more platelet deposition than that induced by subendothelium under the same rheological conditions. A severely damaged vessel wall is a potent inducer of thrombus growth, and inhibition of thrombin significantly reduces platelet accumulation. In addition to collagen, other components of the deep layers of the vessel wall exhibit a potent agonist effect for platelets.

Overall, it is likely that mild injury to the vessel wall, with a limited thrombogenic stimulus, may induce a transient thrombotic mass that, in association with vasoconstriction, may be the underlying cause of the onset of unstable angina. On the other hand, deep vessel injury secondary to severe plaque disruption or ulceration results in the exposure of deep tissue that, in association with high shear conditions and vasoconstriction, may lead to persistent thrombotic occlusion and myocardial infarction.

Spontaneous lysis of a thrombus appears to play a role not only in unstable angina but also in acute myocardial infarction. In both spontaneous and pharmacologic thrombolysis, presence of a residual mural thrombus predisposes to recurrent thrombotic vessel occlusion. First, the residual mural thrombus may protrude into the lumen, resulting in a small residual diameter and, as previously described, an increased local shear rate facilitating platelet activation and deposition in the lesion area. Second, a residual thrombus is a highly thrombogenic surface.

Heparin does not completely inhibit thrombus regrowth after fragmentation or embolization of a thrombus because thrombin is locally available at the thrombus–blood interface to induce rapid regrowth. *In situ* thrombin is not inhibited by systemic heparinization and, in the event of a partial thrombus dislodgement, is a very active local nidus for further platelet activation and acute platelet thrombus formation. It is inhibited by hirudin.

Implications for Treatment

FIRST 6 HOURS

During the first 6 hours following myocardial infarction, the primary management goal is to return coronary blood flow to the affected region. In nontransmural infarction this is frequently not necessary since coronary blood flow to the area usually still exists. Thus the goal is to maintain or improve it. Initial therapy is directed to either relieving coronary spasm or lysing thrombosis. Spasm usually responds to nitroglycerin. Lysis can be accomplished by administration of intravenous or intracoronary arterial (requires left heart catheterization) streptokinase, urokinase, or tissue plasminogen activator (rt-PA). It is clear that full benefits from either technique can only be realized if blood flow is returned quickly. Successful early lytic therapy has been shown to reduce three-week and one-year mortality following infarction in patients with acute anterior wall myocardial infarct.

6 TO 96 HOURS

Patients in whom thrombolytic therapy is initially successful are kept on intra-venous heparin to maintain patency of the coronary artery until coronary arteri-ography can be performed to assess the extent of coronary lesions and determine future therapy. Prevention of recurrent coronary occlusion may involve medical therapy, immediate or delayed coronary angioplasty, or bypass graft surgery, depending on coronary anatomy and left ventricular function.

Other therapeutic agents may also be important in the post-lytic phase of infarctions to maintain coronary artery patency. In addition to heparin, nitrates, or calcium channel blockers may be useful in decreasing coronary vasomotor tone, and aspirin may help prevent platelet plugs from forming. The calcium channel blocker, diltiazem, has been shown to prevent reinfarction and devel-opment of unstable angina during the first 2 weeks following some infarctions. The role of aspirin and other antiplatelet agents in this setting is unclear. Although aspirin has been shown to be an effective treatment for certain patients with unstable angina not associated with acute myocardial infarction, its value in the immediate postinfarction setting, especially with concomitant use of throm-bolytic agents, is currently uncertain.

THROMBOLYTIC THERAPY

Intracoronary administration of streptokinase has been shown to be safe and has been associated with successful reperfusion in 75% of patients with acute myocardial infarction. However, the need for cardiac catheterization and the resultant delay in onset of therapy limits the potential for salvaging ischemic myocardium. Intravenous administration of streptokinase is less successful at reperfusion but still improves ventricular function as well as decreases infarct size and acute mortality when administered within the 4 to 6 hours. The Throm-bosis in Myocardial Infarction (TIMI) trial[26] showed that two-thirds of patients receiving rt-PA had successful reperfusion versus only about one-third of those treated with streptokinase.

To date, thrombolysis has been shown to be effective only during the acute hospital stay. Long-term effects are yet to be determined. However, the incidence of restenosis, despite heparinization in subsequent days and weeks, is high (in the range of 20–30%). No known therapy exists to prevent restenosis, but it generally occurs in patients with 60–80% underlying obstructive plaques. Long-term effects of angioplasty on symptom relief, morbidity, and mortality remain to be determined, particularly since about 30% of patients develop restenosis within 6 to 8 months after angioplasty. Clinical trials are now being performed to assess the long-term effect of angioplasty.

Should non-Q-wave infarction receive thrombolytic therapy considering that early reperfusion probably occurs spontaneously? Angioplasty performed acutely without thrombolytic therapy restores patency in 80–90% of patients, although this approach is not recommended routinely since the unavoidable delay occurring in most cases would jeopardize potential for salvaging myocardium. However, what about the 20–30% of patients who do not undergo reperfusion with thrombolytic therapy? If there were some way to detect these patients within minutes, they would be good candidates for urgent angioplasty. However, to date there are no rapid, objective means for determining whether reperfusion has been successful.

In the future, it is likely that the majority of patients seen within the first 4 to 6 hours of acute myocardial infarction will undergo intravenous thrombolytic therapy with either rt-PA or streptokinase unless there is an obvious contraindication. Both agents will likely be followed by full heparinization for 1 to 2 days, followed by aspirin, 325 mg/day. In many patients, thrombolysis will be followed by cardiac catheterization for consideration of angioplasty in 1 to 2 days. Patients in whom there is residual stenosis of 80% or more in the infarct-related vessel likely will be considered for angioplasty. Indications for surgery are the same as in any patient.

Similarities and Differences in the Myocardial Infarction and Ischemic Stroke Mechanisms

While the pathophysiology and optimal treatment of myocardial infarction are not completely understood, cardiologists are farther along in their understanding of these issues than are neurologists in their understanding of cerebral infarction. From the foregoing discussion, it seems likely that patients with acute myocardial infarction have a high incidence of atherosclerotic plaque rupture which induces local platelet aggregation, increases coronary vasomotor tone, and ultimately precipitates coronary thrombosis. Platelet deposition at the site of arterial injury plays a major role in development of thrombosis and hence the role for antiplatelet agents. When the thrombosis completely occludes the coronary artery, the result often is myocardial infarction. If the thrombus incompletely occludes the artery, or rapidly lyses spontaneously or with therapy, the result is often unstable angina or an infarction that only involves the subendocardium. If the thrombus is small and the coronary artery is large, there may be no clinical sequelae other than fibrotic organization and slow stepwise growth of the plaque.

While the culprit coronary artery lesion at issue in myocardial infarction appears to be the ruptured plaque, there do not appear to be consistent predictors of plaque rupture. Some investigators[21] believe that high-grade pre-existing stenosis at the rupture site is almost always necessary for plaque rupture to lead to significant luminal stenosis and clinical sequelae. However, evidence is accumulating indicating that the degree of coronary artery stenosis does not predict clinical prognosis and that stenoses leading to acute thrombosis and myocardial infarction are <50% in about half of cases, and <70% in two-thirds.[23]

The idea that high-grade stenoses are the dangerous ones is perhaps more consistent with common belief in cerebrovascular disease, i.e. the degree of stenosis correlates directly with the risk of stroke. The European Carotid Surgery Trial (ECST)[10] found that patients with TIA or minor stroke who have a minor stenosis (0–30%) have a very low incidence of stroke. Whereas, both the ECST and North American Symptomatic Carotid Endarterectomy Trial[11] found that similar patients with high-grade stenoses (70–99%) had a very high incidence of ipsilateral cerebral infarction.

Is this apparently important issue of degree of stenosis a *real* difference between MI and stroke? Could it be due to selection bias? Is the finding of mild-to-moderate stenoses causing MI just true for the subset of patients who survive their MI and come to early angiography and thrombolysis? If the difference is real, could it be explained by the size of the arteries involved? Perhaps a small plaque that ruptures and accumulates superimposed thrombus is large enough to occlude the coronary artery and cause infarction, but is not large enough to occlude the larger carotid artery. Further, a high-grade stenosis may be necessary in the carotid artery to create the flow alterations that lead to thrombosis. On the other hand, non-occlusive carotid thrombus probably embolizes and causes distal ischemia; this has been documented in transient monocular blindness. Most likely small emboli also occur in the coronary circulation but are not symptomatic if they fail to cause major arrhythmias, symptomatic myocardial infarct, or sudden death.

Some studies indicate that the composition of the plaque, its morphology, and lipid content may be important, and that the hemodynamic forces to which the plaque is exposed may make it more susceptible to injury. The presence of ulceration, intraplaque hemorrhage, lipid content, and other features in cervical arteries may be detectable and definable in the future by newer sonographic techniques. Thus, our techniques, pathophysiologic concepts and medications remain imperfect but there has been much progress.

References

1. Ordinas A. Presented at the European Stroke Conference, Dusseldorf, Germany, May 1990.
2. Ellis D. Personal communication.
3. Ellis DJ, Roe RL, Bruno JJ, Cranston DJ, McSpadden MM. *Thrombosis and haemostasis.* 1981;**46(1)**:Abstract 543.
4. Gent M, Easton JD, Hachinski VC, et al. The Canadian American ticlopidine study (CATS) in thromboembolic stroke. *Lancet* 1989;**1**:215–220.
5. Hass WK, Easton JD, Adams HP Jr, et al. A randomized trial comparing ticlopidine hydrochloride with aspirin for the prevention of stroke in high-risk patients. *N Engl J Med* 1989;**321**:501–507.
6. Balsano F, Risson P, Viali F, Scrutinio D, et al. Antiplatelet treatment with ticlopidine in unstable angina. *Circulation* 1990;**82**:17–26.

7. FitzGerald GA. Editorial comment: Ticlopidine in unstable angina—A more expensive aspirin? *Circulation* 1990;**82**:296–298.

8. Warlow CP. Editorial: Ticlopidine: a new antithrombotic drug; but is it better than aspirin for long-term use? *J Neurol Neursurg Psychiat* 1990;**53**:185–187.

9. Hunt JR. The role of the carotid arteries in the causation of vascular lesions of the brain with remarks on certain special features of the symptomatology. *Am J Med Sci* 1914;**147**:704–713.

10. North American Symptomatic Carotid Endarterectomy Collaborators. Beneficial effect of carotid endarterectomy in symptomatic patients with high grade stenosis. *N Engl J Med* 1991;**325**:445–453.

11. European Carotid Surgery Trialists. Collaborative Group MRC European Carotid Surgery Trial: Interim results for symptomatic patients with severe (70–99%) or with mild (0–29%) carotid stenosis. *Lancet* 1991;**337**:1235–1243.

12. Hicks SP, Warren S. Infarction of the brain without thrombosis. *AMA Arch Path* 1951;**52**:403–412.

13. Yates PO, Hutchinson EC. Cerebral infarction: the role of the extracranial arteries. Special Report Series No. 33, Medical Research Council, London, HM Stationery Office 1961;**33**:1–95.

14. Hass WK, Fields WS, North RR, Kricheff II, et al. Joint Study of Extracranial Arterial Occlusion. II Arteriography, sites and complications. *JAMA* 1968;**203**:961–968.

15. Dalal PM, Shah PM, Aiyar RR. Arteriographic study of cerebral embolism. *Lancet* 1965;**2**:358–361.

16. Fisher CM. Observations of the fundus oculi in transient monocular blindness. *Neurology* 1959;**9**:333–347.

17. Ross RW. Observations of the retinal blood vessels in monocular blindness. *Lancet* 1961;**2**:1422–1428.

18. Fieschi C, Argentina C, Lenzi GL, Sacchetti ML, et al. Clinical and instrumental evaluation of patients with ischemic stroke within the first six hours. *J Neurol Sci* 1989;**91**:311–322.

19. Sacco RL, Ellenberg JH, Mohr JP, Tatemichi TK, et al. Infarcts of undetermined cause: the NINCDS Stroke Data Bank. *Ann Neurol* 1989;**25**:382–390.

20. Hier DB, Gorelick PB, Mohr JP, Price TR, et al. Stroke recurrence within 2 years after ischemic infarction. *Stroke* 1991;**22**:155–161.

21. Falk E. Morphologic features of unstable atherothrombotic plaques underlying acute coronary syndromes. *Am J Cardiol* 1989;**63**:114E–120E.

22. Mandelkorn JB, Wolf NM, Singh S, Shecter JA, Kersh RI, Rodgers DM, Workman MB, Bentivoglio LG, LaPorte SM, Meister SG. Intracoronary thrombus in nontransmural myocardial infarction and in unstable angina pectoris. *Am J Cardiol* 1983;**52**:1–6.

23. Fuster V, Badimon L, Badimon JJ, Chesebro JH. The pathogenesis of coronary artery disease and the acute coronary syndromes. *N Engl J Med* 1992;**326**:242–250 and 310–318.

24. Fuster V, Stein B, Ambrose JA, Badimon L, Badimon JJ, Chesebro JH. Atherosclerotic plaque rupture and thrombosis. Evolving concepts. *Circulation* 1990;**82**(suppl II): II-47–II-59.

25. Badimon L, Badimon JJ, Cohen M. Chesebro JH, Fuster V. Vessel wall-related risk factors in acute vascular events. *Drugs* 1991, sup:1–9.

26. Chesebro JH, Knatterud G, Roberts R, Borer J, Cohen LS, Dalen J, et al. Thrombolysis in myocardial infarction (TIMI) trial, phase I: A comparison between intravenous tissue plasminogen activator and intravenous streptokinase. *Circulation* 1987;**76**(no.1):142–154.

2
Overview of Ticlopidine's Development

EDOUARD PANAK and MONIQUE VERRY

The discovery and development of a new molecule imply the interplay of chance, audacity, and challenge, as well as lessons from failures and difficulties in reaching scientific and medical recognition of therapeutic progress. Persistent efforts and a consistent preclinical and clinical program should sustain the 10- to 15-year endeavor needed for establishment of a major drug—in this case a drug for cerebro- and cardiovascular event prevention. Ticlopidine's history gives an example of the international cooperation needed between chemists, biologists, pharmacologists, multidisciplinary clinicians, biostatisticians, and health authorities to make progress within the boundaries defined by science and ethics.

It all started in the early 1970s with an unsuccessful effort to find more active and better-tolerated antiinflammatory agents. In the process a small team, from what is now the Sanofi group, synthesized a new series of thienopyridine derivatives and identified their exclusive impact on platelet aggregation at a time when the role of platelets in the genesis of arterial thrombosis had just been suggested. The discovery of aspirin's impact on platelets by Weiss in 1967,[1] together with promising data from several retrospective surveys in aspirin-treated patients, made the concept of antiaggregating agents emerge as a possible therapeutic approach. Rheumatic patients receiving aspirin were reported to exhibit a reduced incidence of myocardial infarction, and concurrently, a protection of coronary and cerebral thrombosis was observed in an 8000-man cohort compared with historical controls.[2] These results kindled the need to scientifically investigate the clinical consequences of antiplatelet action, and thus, several large-scale prospective trials (CDPA, PARIS, AMIS, RRCPE) were initiated.

Researchers from the French Castaigne pharmaceutical company (subsequently integrated into Sanofi) shared the belief that inhibition of platelet function could provide an interesting alternative to oral anticoagulation, which was associated with disappointing efficacy, hemorrhagic side effects, and practical inconvenience. Therefore the scientists included Born's test for platelet aggregation measurement in their systematic screening of new compounds. *Ex vivo* assays with samples from previously treated animals were preferred over *in vitro* tests on animal or human platelet-rich plasma. The only property found for ticlopidine and a few other molecules was inhibition of ADP-induced aggregation after oral administration in rats. It is noteworthy that had ticlopidine been studied only *in vitro* as was usual at that time for the few pharmaceutical companies investigating platelet inhibition, its activity probably would never have been identified since ticlopidine is only weakly active *in vitro* and requires metabolism before its interaction with platelets.

Three further experimental conditions contributed to the discovery of ticlopidine: 1) oral administration, since the drug is inactive intravenously; 2) choosing rats, the most sensitive species among common laboratory animals; and 3) using ADP as the aggregation agonist, which later was revealed to correspond to the drug specificity. Also somewhat fortuitous was the selection of ticlopidine instead of competitive candidates exhibiting at least as effective an antithrombotic effect in rat models of arterial thrombosis but which were subsequently found to be ineffective in humans.

At the beginning, ticlopidine researchers were faced with the problem of generating a development strategy for a purely antiplatelet drug that was clearly devoid of any other pharmacoclinical activities. This was a difficult task in the absence of reference clinical guidelines in the field—no trial had yet demonstrated the efficacy of aspirin as an antithrombotic drug. This led to the conception of a four-step, sequential clinical scheme, with the eventual objective of clinically validating the concept that an antiplatelet agent could reduce morbidity and mortality resulting from cardiovascular and cerebrovascular diseases.

The first step was to confirm ticlopidine's antiplatelet activity in humans. This was first done in healthy volunteers and later in patients with cerebrovascular, coronary, and peripheral vascular disease as soon as allowed by animal safety studies. These data documented the broad spectrum of ticlopidine's antiplatelet properties that had already been observed in animal pharmacology studies. Ticlopidine inhibits primary and secondary adenosine diphosphate (ADP) induced aggregation in a dose-dependent manner for repeated daily dosages of 250 mg, 500 mg, 750 mg, and 1000 mg, with a steady state reached between the third and fifth days. After treatment discontinuation, a residual effect persists over seven days, suggesting an irreversible alteration of platelet function by ticlopidine therapy. To a lesser extent, the drug inhibits aggregation induced by collagen, adrenalin, thrombin, and platelet activating factor (PAF). It inhibits the platelet release reaction and prolongs bleeding time. These results kindled researchers' interest in the compound's mode of action, which for a long time remained essentially characterized by its difference from that of classical agents, such as aspirin and non-steroidal anti-inflammatory drugs (NSAIDs), which act through the inhibition of cyclooxygenase. It was later determined that ticlopidine specifically inhibited ADP-dependent activation of the glycoprotein IIb/IIIa (GPIIb/IIIa) platelet receptor for fibrinogen binding, which represents the crucial final step for platelet aggregation to occur whatever the inducer.[3-6] This explained its broad spectrum inhibition as well as the fact that it could be overwhelmed by an agonist excess save for ADP itself.

At the second stage of ticlopidine's development, the methodological problem arose of evaluating the therapeutic effect of an antiaggregating agent in patients. By this stage health authorities in various countries had set up clear regulatory rules, specifying that the pharmacological activity of a drug in patients was insufficient to claim its subsequent benefit, and that its therapeutic usefulness had to be clinically and statistically demonstrated in order to obtain registration for the relevant indications.

Considering the potential benefits of ticlopidine, long-term toxicology and oncogenicity studies were undertaken early according to international guidelines. The technical impracticability of therapeutic dose-ranging trials with antiplatelet agents (which raises the question of optimal daily dose for aspirin) led researchers to consider that a daily dosage of 500 mg, which was generally well tolerated (whereas doses of 750 mg or more would cause gastric upset or diarrhea in a large proportion of patients) and elicited a submaximal inhibition of ADP-induced platelet aggregation (about 50% with 2 mol/l), could be appropriate in ensuring a protective effect against occurrence or recurrence of thromboembolic disorders.

It was then decided to conduct short-term trials in conditions of systematically increased platelet activation (extracorporeal circulation in heart surgery and chronic hemodialysis). The correction induced by ticlopidine on platelet count depression in cardiopulmonary bypass and of platelet microaggregate deposition on dialyzer membranes could be documented as significant in studies with small numbers of patients. This resulted in obtaining the first marketing approvals as well as generating a first validation of the dose selection for the respective indications.

At this stage, the clinical development of ticlopidine also had to take into account the issue of preventative therapies for thromboembolic diseases beyond the control of risk factors. Unlike potentially curative situations, the objective is not to define a success ratio on a 100%-affected patient group but to follow up two cohorts of comparable patients with an approximately known risk of critical events in the expectation of documenting a given relative risk reduction.

In the early 1980s the third step was expansion of the program to confirm the drug's efficacy during medium-term clinical trials of limited size.[5] The initial approach was set up to evaluate ticlopidine's benefit in selected high-risk patients. Epidemiological information concerning the incidence of thrombotic outcomes in the population with the disease of interest was needed to calculate the sample size of patients required in order to demonstrate a statistically significant difference between the treated group and the control group: the lower the frequency of critical events selected, the higher the number of patients required.

At this point in ticlopidine's development resting on a scarcely-validated concept, the company and its partners had to focus on the more cost-effective clinical investments. Therefore, the objective of early trials was to search for: 1) patency maintenance of access sites in patients on chronic hemodialysis; 2) patency maintenance of coronary artery bypass grafts; and 3) prevention of ischemic strokes in patients treated by surgery after subarachnoid hemorrhage.

Concurrently, another approach focused on assessing the improvement or stabilization of thrombotic clinical situations in the hope of finding a model in which platelet inhibition would result in symptomatic improvement of some sort. This part of the approach included: 1) treatment of ischemic ulcers due to arterial occlusion; 2) improvement of visual acuity after retinal vein occlusion; 3) prevention of vasculo-occlusive crisis in Raynaud's syndrome and in sickle cell disease (the latter in relation to the additional effects of ticlopidine on red cell deformability and blood viscosity); and 4) peripheral vascular disease.

Globally, ticlopidine exerted beneficial effects in patients undergoing hemodialysis or coronary surgery, suffering from ischemic leg ulcers, experiencing subarachnoid hemorrhage, and complaining of intermittent claudication.

In 107 patients undergoing maintenance hemodialysis and subject to repetitive thrombotic episodes, ticlopidine significantly reduced (by half, in comparison with placebo) the incidence of occlusions of arteriovenous shunts or fistulas and reduced the frequency of surgery for removal of clots or reconstruction for blood access while improving dialysis performance.[6] Ticlopidine showed a similar efficacy against placebo in primary prevention of occlusion of vascular access sites when initiated before shunt placement in 169 patients enrolled in four double-blind studies.[7-10]

The benefit of coronary bypass grafts in patients suffering from severe coronary ischemia is limited by the risk of graft occlusion, which affects about 15% of patients in the first month and about 30% within the first year as described in Chapter 7 of this book. In a controlled study of anticoagulants in 166 patients undergoing aortocoronary bypass grafts and receiving either ticlopidine or nicoumalone (prothrombin time 20–25%) on the first postoperative day, the graft patency rates were higher in the ticlopidine group (64%) than in the nicoumalone group (58%).[11] In a placebo-controlled trial involving 173 patients followed for 1 year, ticlopidine (started the second postoperative day) significantly reduced the graft occlusion rate on day 10 (7.1% vs. 13.4%, p = 0.05), on day 180 (15% vs. 24%, p = 0.02), and on day 360 (15.9% vs. 26.1%, p = 0.001). When one considers individual grafts (i.e., grafts to only one coronary), the occlusion rate was significantly, about 50%, lower (p = 0.01) in the ticlopidine group than in the placebo group: day 10—5.4% vs. 15.8%, day 180—11.2% vs. 25.2%, and day 360—12.6% vs. 26.6%.[12] Favorable results in the CABG studies were recorded in spite of the trialists' reluctance to start treatment preoperatively, a therapeutic attitude perceived as likely to maximize efficacy but also to entail an added hemorrhagic risk.

Two double-blind, placebo-controlled studies,[13-16] in about 200 patients with chronic arterial occlusion due to arteriosclerosis obliterans or thromboangiitis obliterans who were followed for short periods of 1 to 2 months, demonstrated a significant benefit of ticlopidine. Ticlopidine treatment produced complete healing or marked improvement of ulcers by stimulating epithelialization and local revascularization. Ticlopidine also has been shown to retard the progression of atherosclerosis in a placebo-controlled trial involving 43 patients with arterial obstruction of the legs followed for 1 year. Serial arteriography of the lower limbs was performed at the beginning of the study and at 1 year. Angiograms were analyzed with a scoring system based on the severity and length of stenosis. Atherosclerotic plaque progression was significantly less marked in the ticlopidine-treated patients: 95% stabilization of atherosclerotic lesions in the ticlopidine group compared with 37% deterioration in the placebo group.[15]

Several double-blind, placebo-controlled trials were conducted with ticlopidine in patients who were suffering from chronic intermittent claudication due to obstructive peripheral vascular disease in a further attempt to assess the effects of ticlopidine on functional symptomatology. The two largest studies, 169 and 203 patients respectively, showed an improvement in pain-free and/or maximum walking distance in the ticlopidine groups as compared with placebo, and more important, the systematic recording of cardiovascular events demonstrated a two-thirds reduction in these outcomes, indicating the drug's beneficial effect in prevention of vascular complications related to atherosclerosis.[16-17]

As early as 1986 short-term portions of a program of studies on peripheral vascular disease of the lower limbs demonstrated that ticlopidine significantly reduced fatal or nonfatal ischemic peripheral and cerebrovascular accidents by two-thirds compared to placebo (3% in the ticlopidine group, 9% in the placebo group) in patients suffering from intermittent claudication. This was shown using meta-analysis of four similar studies involving more than 600 patients followed from 6 months to 1 year.[18] In 1986 these data led to the extension of indications for ticlopidine in France for the prevention of cerebral and peripheral ischemic complications in patients with atherosclerotic intermittent claudication. Further approvals were granted by other European health authorities in the following years.

In view of these findings, the results of a larger and long-term, placebo-controlled trial in claudicants started in 1980, the Swedish Ticlopidine Multicentre Study (STIMS)[19] extensively described in Chapter 6 were eagerly awaited to further define the role of ticlopidine in prevention of thrombotic cardiovascular events in that patient population.

Occurring at the same time as these studies in the cerebral vascular disease field was the double-blind Japanese ticlopidine study in transient ischemic attacks (TIA) involving 340 patients. This study demonstrated the superiority of ticlopidine over aspirin at 1 year in the incidence of fatal or nonfatal cerebral and myocardial infarctions and the recurrence of TIA. The small number of patients required for this study was related to the selected endpoints—completed thromboembolic events and transient ischemic attacks, the latter being much more frequent than the former and accepted by the local health authorities, in spite of their subjective character, as the basis of the efficacy evaluation.[20] This was of clear interest to the Ticlopidine-Aspirin Stroke Study (TASS)[21] trialists who were halfway through their full-scale study, which was much larger because only "hard endpoints" were considered.

These converging data reinforced the commitment of Sanofi and the ticlopidine trialists to go ahead with the fourth step, which corresponded to the real challenge of documenting the drug's efficacy in the prevention of arterial thrombosis—that is, the prevention of stroke, myocardial infarction, and vascular death. In the field of preventative medicine, a further difficulty arose due to the side effects of the drug, which implied ethical considerations linked to the benefit/risk ratio evaluation. Once the risk of side effects became known, more than 3 years after the initial marketing, Sanofi and its partners decided to set up safety monitoring procedures in clinical trials and for postmarketing surveillance. Ticlopidine's known side effects, which had been reported to health authorities, were continuously documented and their imputability assessed in relation to treatment. The more common adverse effects reported were gastrointestinal disorders (nausea, diarrhea) and skin rashes, but the expanded use of ticlopidine led to identification of new side effects with a low incidence, particularly neutropenias, sometimes severe but most often occurring during the first 3 months of treatment and reversible upon drug discontinuation. This contributed to the company actively choosing to refocus the development program toward diseases associated with a high vascular risk so that a potentially favorable benefit/risk ratio could be reached, notably in the absence of any alternative satisfactory effective treatment.

In the early 1980s, in addition to STIMS,[19] TASS,[21] discussed in Chapter 5, was started in North America along the lines of the Canadian Cooperative Study.[22] The decision was then made to add a program in patients undergoing PTCA (see Chapter 7) and a trial in patients with completed stroke, i.e., the Canadian-American Ticlopidine Study (CATS),[23] in order to assess the drug (Chapter 5). This was undertaken with the expectation that a "reasonable" (i.e., 25–30%) relative risk reduction in patients at high-risk for stroke could result in an absolute risk reduction clearly higher than the expression of potential side effects. Altogether, the long-term program involved more than 5000 patients (including a diabetic retinopathy effort), most of whom were followed from 2 to 7 years.

For protocol design and subsequent evaluation of data, several medical and methodological concerns had to be considered. Key issues included types of patients at risk (here the number of subjects and the duration of follow-up);

Table 2.1. Comparison of characteristics of STIMS, TASS, and CATS studies.

	STIMS	TASS	CATS
Patients	Chronic peripheral arterial disease. Abnormal systolic pressure gradient between upper arm and ankle.	Stroke precursors/ minor stroke	Completed stroke
Intention to treat	All randomized	All randomized	All randomized but "truly ineligible"
Efficacy	All intention to treat within 15 days of drug discontinuation	All intention to treat except ineligibles and within 10 days of drug discontinuation	All intention to treat within 28 days after drug discontinuation
Primary analysis	Intention to treat (2 tailed)	Intention to treat (2 tailed)	Efficacy (1 tailed)
Primary outcome cluster	• Protocol endpoints fatal or nonfatal myocardial infarction and stroke plus TIAs • Study endpoints as above + sudden death	Stroke or death	Ischemic stroke, myocardial infarction (MI), vascular death
Secondary outcome cluster(s)	—	Fatal or nonfatal stroke	• Stroke, MI, death • Fatal or nonfatal stroke • Vascular death • Death
Study size—patient numbers	687 patients ticlopidine: 346 placebo: 341	3069 patients ticlopidine: 1529 placebo: 1540	1072 patients ticlopidine: 531 placebo: 541
Mean follow-up	5.6 years	3.2 years	2 years

choice of control treatment; selection of appropriate outcome events; quality assessment of the trial's overall stages; types of data analysis; and evaluation of the benefit/risk ratio of the study therapy.

First, sample size is a main consideration in a clinical setting where small or large numbers of patients at high risk need to be studied in order to have a high probability of detecting important clinical benefits. This requires knowledge of the natural history of the disease of interest in terms of quantified morbidity and mortality. For cerebrovascular disease, patients with transient ischemic attacks have a 6% annual risk of stroke and death,[24] and aspirin's overall benefit in reducing this incidence had been estimated at 22% within 3 years.[25] In order to demonstrate ticlopidine's superiority over aspirin with 90% power, calculations showed that 3000 patients with an average 3-year follow-up had to be enrolled.

Second, the choice of the control treatment, placebo or a drug clearly recognized as active, addressed questions of ethics and the appropriate dose regimen for aspirin. For stroke survivors, aspirin was unwarranted because its effects had not been documented in that population. Therefore, placebo was used as a control agent in CATS. Similarly, as there was no experience with antiplatelet agents in patients with peripheral arterial disease for the reduction of systemic thrombotic events, placebo was used as the control in STIMS whose patients were however subjected to vigorous control of risk factors. A placebo-controlled study raises the problem of intermediate statistical analyses, which lower the power of the trial and, as such, might deprive patients of a new active drug but may be mandatory for ethical reasons. The current controversy, involving aspirin's optimal low dose, had not yet emerged in the early 1980s, so the approved American and Canadian dose of 1300 mg aspirin/day was chosen for comparison with ticlopidine for study of primary stroke prevention in patients suffering from TIA or minor stroke.

Third, researchers had to choose the most relevant outcomes to the natural history of the disease. The risk of these outcomes also needed to be potentially reduced by antiplatelet therapy, and consequently, to be the most suitable for evaluating the treatment's protective effect on the occurrence or recurrence of serious vascular events. Analyses should be based on actuarial methods that record time to first event among those considered, i.e., fatal or nonfatal stroke, myocardial infarction, vascular death, sudden death, and death from any cause. The primary criteria for analysis were different in the STIMS, TASS, and CATS studies. Composite endpoints in STIMS included fatal or nonfatal stroke and myocardial infarction, as well as occurrence of severe or recurrent TIAs. The primary outcomes selected in TASS were stroke or death from any cause, as in the previous Canadian Cooperative trial,[22] with secondary outcomes of fatal or nonfatal stroke.

While these primary clusters would appear reasonable, a more relevant cluster (i.e., stroke, myocardial infarction, and vascular death), chosen in the CATS study after completed stroke, is now suggested as the most representative for analysis or meta-analysis of antiplatelet therapy in the prevention of ischemic vascular events. This latter cluster has the advantage of including the three major clinical outcomes relatively common in ischemic patients and likely to be influenced by antiplatelet agents, whereas nonvascular death is unlikely to be altered by such drugs. Hence, this composite outcome tends to increase the number of salient critical events in the control group as compared to target-organ-specific subsets, such as MI plus cardiac death in ischemic heart disease, and makes it easier to demonstrate a true overall benefit of the anti-platelet treatment. Consequently, this approach should reduce sample size requirements for reaching statistical significance. Indeed, it has worked for the CATS program, together with the advantage of the placebo control, allowing the study to be conducted on the basis of about 1000 patients with an average follow-up of 2 years.

Fourth, beyond quality of design, trials needed to be conducted with rigor and discipline so that valid results could be obtained. Quality assessment of the protocols, trials, and data required specific organization with several scientific and coordinating units, as well as a predefined method of analysis to avoid bias in estimating potential therapeutic benefit and to guarantee the trial's integrity. The large-scale prospective trials were organized around central committees: a steering committee having overall responsibility for the study and resolving policy issues encountered during the course of the study; a body to adjudicate qualifying events and outcomes; and an independent safety committee, privy to the randomization code, guaranteeing the ethics of the trial and safety of the patients. These committees worked in close proximity to operational coordination centers. The latter ensured compliance with good clinical practice, notably approval of the protocols by ethics committees and patient-informed consent recording, and they also collected, validated, and updated data forwarded to statisticians for interim and final analyses.

Fifth, methodological concerns that were raised about analyses of such trials were usually reported in two ways, taking into account predefined stratification of the patients to be enrolled. Intention-to-treat analysis includes all outcome events in all the patients randomized (even if they are later deemed ineligible as not conforming to inclusion criteria, are withdrawn for any reason or are not compliant with the therapy). It does not incorporate bias, but it can induce a marked loss in sensitivity regarding beneficial effects of the drug because of the "noise" introduced by protocol deviations. Another strategy, efficacy analysis, assesses the results only in eligible patients in whom the outcome events occur while on treatment. This yields information about the expected effect of the drug, but the same degree of benefit should not necessarily be expected in a treated general population.

It is to be noted that the operational definitions of all these seemingly simple terms were not totally identical across the three studies, reflecting various successive approaches in the field of clinical trial methodology. Indeed, all the above issues were taken carefully into consideration by the three groups of investigators between 1978 and 1983, in a time period when methodological issues were eagerly debated on the occasion of each of the many trials reaching completion as well as those being initiated. As a consequence of this shifting scientific background, the three studies were undertaken with minor departures from each other in design, as shown above in Table 2.1.

Finally, after completion of the trials (which are described in other chapters), one of the main issues to be considered in result analysis was evaluation of the benefit/risk ratio of ticlopidine in the prevention of arterial thrombotic processes considering three aspects:

- The risks of vascular disease.
- The drug's benefit in reducing these risks and its value over existing therapies.
- The risk in relation to ticlopidine treatment and the possibility of controlling its clinical consequences by appropriate surveillance procedures.

Based on these findings, a first registration of ticlopidine for prevention of arterial thrombotic complications (stroke, myocardial infarction, sudden deaths from vascular origin) after a first atherosclerosis-related ischemic cerebral event was granted by the French health authorities in October 1990. In April 1991, the Health Protection Branch (HPB) granted approval of ticlopidine in Canada as first-line therapy in all patients at high risk of stroke, including both men and women and those at risk of both first and recurrent stroke, with the requirement that close monitoring should be performed for potential side effects during the first 3 months of treatment. In November 1991, the Food and Drug Administration (FDA) granted approval of ticlopidine in the USA to "reduce the risk of thrombotic stroke (fatal or nonfatal) in patients who have experienced stroke precursors, and in patients who have had a completed thrombotic stroke, who are intolerant to aspirin therapy where indicated to prevent stroke." Recommendations for patient monitoring require blood cell counts and white cell differentials every 2 weeks during the first 3 months.

When reflecting on the sequence of events in ticlopidine's development process and considering the impracticability of therapeutic dose-ranging trials and the eventual need for assessing a delicate benefit-to-risk balance, which might be dependent on the dose selected, it might be necessary to question the appropriateness of the initial dosage. The initial biological dose response study was reconducted in North America on a fairly large scale in elderly healthy volunteers[26] and confirmed that a daily dose of 500 mg was an optimal dosage while larger doses, up to 750 mg, would produce only minimal additional biological effects at the cost of lesser clinical tolerance. Converging information was generated by a French study in early diabetic retinopathy (TIMAD),[27] in which the effects of ticlopidine on retinal microaneurysm progression were assessed over 3 years versus placebo and in which platelet aggregation was used to estimate compliance as well as long-term maintenance of platelet effects (with due precautions to avoid unblinding the trial). This data indicated that there was a linear correlation between clinical efficacy, as documented by a reduced rate of increase of microaneurysm counts and the extent of inhibition of aggregation elicited.

The developments in peripheral arterial disease and in TIA/minor stroke patients should stimulate a thoughtful search for further compounds, because in both instances conclusions from "softer" endpoints (including peripheral vascular surgery on the one hand, occurrence of TIAs on the other) and more limited patient numbers and exposure had heralded the findings of the large scale "definitive studies." Nevertheless the data from STIMS, TASS, and CATS, and the documented effectiveness in preventing major clinical outcomes provide key elements to enter into the benefit/risk evaluation.

Currently, ticlopidine appears to be the reference drug for prevention of vascular complications in patients suffering from intermittent claudication or after a completed stroke, as well as a better agent than aspirin for secondary prevention after minor ischemic cerebral attacks.

Ticlopidine is now internationally recognized for its efficacy as a major drug that will help protect patients at high vascular risk against thousands of fatal or nonfatal occlusive events each year. Beyond the improved vascular prognosis that ticlopidine should provide to many patients, its already long scientific and clinical history has also demonstrated its usefulness as a biological and therapeutic tool to better understand the role of platelets in the mechanisms of arterial thrombosis.

References

1. Weiss HJ, Aledort LM. Impaired platelet/connective tissue reaction after aspirin ingestion. *Lancet* 1967;**2**:495–497.
2. Craven LL. Prevention of coronary and cerebral thrombosis. *Miss Valley Med J* 1956;**78**:213–215.
3. Saltiel E, Ward A. Ticlopidine. A review of its pharmacodynamic and pharmacokinetic properties, and therapeutic efficacy in platelet-dependent disease states. *Drugs* 1987; **34**:222–262.
4. McTavish D, Faulds D, Goa KL. Ticlopidine. An updated review of its pharmacology and therapeutic use in platelet-dependent disorders. *Drugs* 1990;**40(2)**:238–259.
5. Panak EA, Maffrand JP, Picard-Fraire C, Vallée E, Blanchard JF, Roncucci R. Ticlopidine: a promise for the prevention and treatment of thrombosis and its complications. *Haemostasis* 1983;**31**(suppl 1):1–54.
6. Kobayashi K, Maeda K, Koshikawa S, Kawaguchi Y, Shimizu N, et al. Antithrombotic therapy with ticlopidine in chronic renal failure patients on maintenance hemodialysis— a multicenter collaborative double blind study. *Thromb Res* 1980;**30**:255–261.
7. Ell S, Mihindukulasuriya JCL, O'Brien JR, Polak A, Vernham G. Ticlopidine in the prevention of blockage of fistulae and shunts. Abstract 332 from the 7th International Congress on Thrombosis, Valencia, Spain, 1982, October 13–16, p 180.
8. Fiskerstrand CE, Thompson IW, Burnet ME, Williams P, Anderton JL. Double-blind randomized trial of the effects of ticlopidine in arteriovenous fistulas for hemodialysis. *Artificial Organs* 1985;**9**:61–63.

9. Grontoft KC, Mulec H, Gutierrez A, Olander R. Thromboprophylactic effect of ticlopidine in arteriovenous fistulas for hemodialysis. *Scand J Urol and Nephrol* 1985;**19**: 55–57.

10. Panak EA, Blanchard JF, Roe RL. Evaluation of the antithrombotic efficacy of ticlopidine in man. *Agents and Actions Suppl*, Ticlopidine: Quo Vadis? 1984;**15**:148–166.

11. Rothlin ME, Pfluger N, Speiser K, Goebels N, Krayenbuhl HP, et al. Platelet inhibitors versus anticoagulants for prevention of aorto-coronary bypass graft occlusion. *Eur Heart J* 1985;**6**:168–175.

12. Limet R, David JL, Magotteaux P, Larock MP, Rigo P. Prevention of aortocoronary bypass occlusion: beneficial effect of ticlopidine on early and late patency rates of venous coronary bypass grafts—a double-blind study. *J Thorac Cardiovasc Surg* 1987;**94**:773–783.

13. Katsumura T, Mishima Y, Kamiya K, Sakaguchi S, Tanabe T, et al. Therapeutic effect of ticlopidine, a new inhibitor of platelet aggregation, on chronic arterial occlusive diseases, a double-blind study, versus placebo. *Angiology* 1982;**33**:357–367.

14. Bourde C, Eschwège E, Verry M. Controlled clinical trial of an antiaggregating agent, ticlopidine, in vascular ulcers of the leg. Abstract 0271. *Thromb Haemost* 1981;**46**:91.

15. Stiegler H, Hess H, Mietaschk A, Tramppisch HJ, Ingrisch H. Einfluss von ticlopidin auf die perifere obliterierende arteriopathie. *Deutsche Medizinische Wochenschrift* 1984;**109**:1240–1243.

16. Arcan JC, Blanchard JF, Boissel JP, Destors JM, Panak EA. Multicenter double-blind study of ticlopidine in the treatment of intermittent claudication and the prevention of its complications. *Angiology* 1988;**39(9)**:802–811.

17. Ellis DJ. Treatment of intermittent claudication with ticlopidine. Abstract, 32nd annual meeting of the International Committee on Thrombosis and Haemostasis and the 9th Congress of the Mediterranean League against Thromboembolic Diseases. Jerusalem, 1986, June 1–6.

18. Boissel JP, Peyrieux JC, Destors JM. Is it possible to reduce the risk of cardiovascular events in subjects suffering from intermittent claudication of the lower limbs? *Thromb Haemost* 1989;**62(2)**:681–685.

19. Janzon L, Bergqvist D, Boberg J, Boberg M, Eriksson I, Lindgarde F, Persson G. Prevention of myocardial infarction and stroke in patients with intermittent claudication: effects of ticlopidine. Results from STIMS, the Swedish Ticlopidine Multicentre Study. *J Int Med* 1990;**227**:301–308.

20. Tohgi H, Murakami M. The effect of ticlopidine on TIA compared with aspirin: a double-blind, twelve-month follow-up study and open 24-month follow-up study. *Jpn J Med* 1987;**26**:117–119.

21. Hass WK, Easton JD, Adams HP, et al. for the Ticlopidine Aspirin Stroke Study Group. A randomized trial comparing ticlopidine hydrochloride with aspirin for the prevention of stroke in high-risk patients. *N Engl J Med* 1989;**321**:501–507.

22. Canadian Cooperative Study Group: a randomized trial of aspirin and sulfinpyrazone in threatened stroke. *N Engl J Med* 1978;**299**:53–59.

23. Gent M, Easton JD, Hachinski VC, et al. and the CATS Group. The Canadian American Ticlopidine Study (CATS) in thromboembolic stroke. *Lancet* 1989;June 3:1215–1220.

24. Dennis MS, Bamford JM, Sandercock PAG, Warlow CP. Prognosis of transient ischemic attacks in the Oxfordshire Community Stroke Project. *Stroke* 1990;**21**:848–853.

25. Antiplatelet Trialists' Collaboration. Secondary prevention of vascular disease by pro-
    longed antiplatelet treatment. *Br Med J* 1988;**296**:320–331.
26. Data on file.
27. TIMAD Study Group. Ticlopidine treatment reduces the progression of nonproliferative
    diabetic retinopathy. *Arch Ophthal* 1990;**108**:1577–1583.

3
Pharmacodynamics and Pharmacokinetics of Ticlopidine

PHILIP TEITELBAUM

Introduction

Ticlopidine is a unique inhibitor of platelet aggregation. It has, therefore, been evaluated extensively during the past several years for prevention of disease in which undesirable thromboembolism is thought to play a role. Mechanistically, ticlopidine is different from other types of platelet aggregation inhibitors and may be thought of as a "broad spectrum" inhibitor of platelet function in that it inhibits platelet aggregation mediated by several interdependent pathways of activation. Oral administration of ticlopidine to humans results in *ex vivo* inhibition of platelet aggregation in response to a number of inducers, including ADP, thrombin, collagen, serotonin, arachidonic acid, epinephrine, and platelet activating factor.[1] Ticlopidine appears to act at a final common pathway for platelet activation, which involves an ADP-induced conformational modification of the platelet membrane glycoprotein (GPIIb/IIIa) to form the fibrinogen binding site. The observed effects of ticlopidine on several inducers of platelet aggregation may all result from blockade of the amplifying effect of endogenous ADP released from platelet-dense granules.[2] The precise mechanism by which ticlopidine inhibits the effect of ADP on activation of the platelet membrane glycoprotein has not been defined (see Chapter 4 for a complete discussion of ticlopidine's mechanism of action).

Ticlopidine's effects on ADP-induced aggregation are more pronounced and reproducible than those observed for other inducers of platelet aggregation. As a result, *ex vivo* inhibition of ADP-induced activation of platelets, determined by Born's[3] method, is the most frequently monitored parameter in pharmacodynamic studies of ticlopidine. Following treatment with ticlopidine, platelet rich plasma (PRP) is prepared from anticoagulated blood by low speed centrifugation. Various concentrations of ADP are added to the PRP, and ADP-induced aggregation is quantitated by measuring the increase in optical transmission that occurs when the platelets in PRP aggregate. It must be emphasized that this method for quantitating ticlopidine's inhibitory effect is based entirely on *in vitro* laboratory measurement and must not be confused with quantitation of ticlopidine's actual therapeutic effect in preventing thromboembolic disease.

The relationship between laboratory measurements of the extent of platelet function inhibition and ticlopidine's efficacy in preventing thromboembolic disease is not well defined.

Characterization of ticlopidine's pharmacokinetic properties must also be qualified. After chronic dosing ticlopidine is the predominant circulating drug-related component in plasma (see below), and essentially all studies of ticlopidine's pharmacokinetics in humans involve quantitation of ticlopidine in plasma, usually by gas chromatography. When added to PRP at concentrations that circulate in plasma following therapeutic doses, ticlopidine is essentially inactive as an inhibitor of platelet aggregation.[4,5] Ticlopidine's lack of direct inhibitory activity has resulted in speculation that metabolic activation of ticlopidine is integral to its mechanism of action, but to date, the exact role of metabolism in ticlopidine's platelet inhibitory activity is unclear. Evidence obtained from studies in which plasma from subjects treated with ticlopidine is mixed with platelets from control subjects demonstrates the absence of circulating moieties that directly inhibit platelet aggregation (see Chapter 4). To date only a single metabolite of ticlopidine, 2-hydroxy ticlopidine, has been demonstrated to possess significant platelet inhibitory activity.[6,7] However, this metabolite has not been found circulating in plasma. Like ticlopidine, 2-hydroxy ticlopidine is inactive *in vitro* and is only active after *in vivo* administration in animals. Because it is ticlopidine that either directly or indirectly inhibits platelet function, and because ticlopidine is the predominant drug-related moiety in plasma, concentrations of ticlopidine in plasma have been utilized to define its pharmacokinetics.

A number of studies in animals have been performed to characterize the pharmacodynamics and metabolic disposition of ticlopidine following administration by different routes and according to different dosing regimens. For the most part, these data corroborate results of numerous pharmacodynamic and pharmacokinetic studies with ticlopidine in humans. Discussion of pharmacodynamics and pharmacokinetics of ticlopidine in this chapter will focus on results of studies conducted in humans. Pharmacokinetic and pharmacodynamic properties of ticlopidine in both animals and humans have been reviewed previously.[1,8,9]

Absorption, Metabolism, and Excretion

Administration of single oral doses of [^{14}C]-ticlopidine to volunteers[10-12] results in rapid absorption of radioactivity into the systemic circulation, with peak levels in plasma occurring within 1.5 hours after dosing (Figure 3.1). Ticlopidine's extent of absorption and oral bioavailability in humans has not been directly quantified, in part because parenteral doses have not been administered to humans. Studies in several animal species with oral and intravenous doses of [^{14}C]-ticlopidine have shown that ticlopidine is completely absorbed.[13] Based on data in humans that indicate approximately 60% of an oral dose of [^{14}C]-ticlopidine is recovered in the urine[11,12] and only low levels of intact ticlopidine

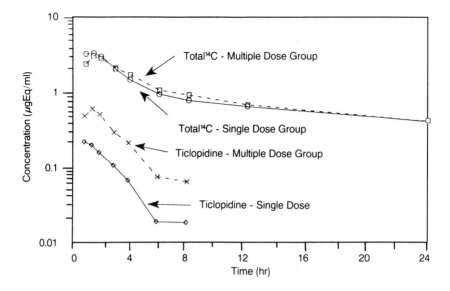

FIGURE 3.1. Concentrations of radioactivity and [^{14}C]-ticlopidine in the plasma of subjects given a single dose of [^{14}C]-ticlopidine alone or after treatment with 250 mg bid nonlabeled ticlopidine for 10 days. Data are the mean values for four subjects in each group (Syntex).

are recovered in feces, oral absorption of ticlopidine in humans is also estimated to be complete.

Following administration of [^{14}C]-ticlopidine to humans, most of the radioactivity in blood is found in the plasma fraction. Although the principal pharmacologic effect of ticlopidine is inhibition of platelet aggregation, radioactivity has not been detected in association with platelets in humans given [^{14}C]-ticlopidine or in rats given much higher doses of high-specific-activity, tritiated ticlopidine.[10-12]

The profile of radioactivity in plasma following administration of a single 250 mg dose of [^{14}C]-ticlopidine was determined in untreated subjects and subjects pretreated with nonlabeled ticlopidine at a dose of 250 mg bid for 10 days.[12] In untreated subjects, ticlopidine accounts for only 5% of AUC for plasma radioactivity during the first 8 hours after administration (Figure 3.1). Similar results were found following a single 750 mg dose of [^{14}C]-ticlopidine.[10] Numerous unidentified metabolites are present in plasma. After multiple dosing with nonlabeled ticlopidine, the proportion of ticlopidine to total radioactivity in plasma increases such that ticlopidine is the major circulating component in plasma and accounts for approximately 15% of plasma radioactivity through 8 hours. The increase in ticlopidine concentrations and the increased proportion of total radioactivity after multiple dosing suggests that metabolism of ticlopidine

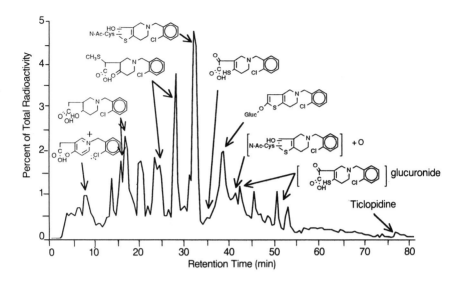

FIGURE 3.2. Profile of metabolites present in urine of subjects given a single 250 mg oral dose of [^{14}C]-ticlopidine. Structures represent tentative assignments based on liquid chromatography/mass-spectrometric analysis (Syntex).

is saturated after chronic dosing. This finding is consistent with multiple-dose pharmacokinetic studies of ticlopidine.[14]

Ticlopidine binds reversibly to plasma proteins, mainly to serum albumin and lipoproteins, and this binding is nonsaturable over the range of concentrations that occur after therapeutic doses.[15] Approximately 15% of ticlopidine in plasma is bound to α_1-acid glycoprotein. In addition to reversibly binding to plasma proteins, significant levels of ticlopidine-associated radioactivity in plasma are irreversibly bound to plasma proteins.[12] One hour after a single 250 mg oral dose of [^{14}C]-ticlopidine, an average of 0.20 µgEq/ml of radioactivity (6% of total radioactivity in plasma) is covalently bound to plasma proteins, and the levels increase slowly until reaching an average maximal concentration of 0.35 µgEq/ml after approximately 15 hours. From 24 hours onward, radioactivity irreversibly bound to protein accounts for most radioactivity in plasma. Levels of radioactivity irreversibly bound to plasma proteins decrease slowly, with a terminal half-life of 3–5 days. While the mechanism for formation of ticlopidine-protein adducts has not been defined, metabolism of ticlopidine to 2-hydroxy ticlopidine may be involved. Incubation of this metabolite with plasma proteins indicates that 2-hydroxy ticlopidine nonenzymatically reacts with proteins, probably by acylation, to form covalent adducts.[13] It is not known whether this phenomenon (ticlopidine's irreversible binding to proteins) plays a role in ticlopidine's

TABLE 3.1. Pharmacokinetic parameters of ticlopidine in young and elderly subjects given 250 mg bid for 21 days.

Parameter	Young	Elderly	p-value
Day 1			
n	12	13	
Cmax (µg/ml)	0.41 (0.24)	0.70 (0.52)	0.035
Tmax (h)	2.0 (1.0-3.0)	2.0 (1.0-4.0)	ns
$T_{1/2}$ (h)	7.9 (3.0)	12.7 (0.9)	0.013
AUC (µg•h/ml)	1.4 (0-0.8)	2.8 (1.2)	0.002
Day 21			
n	12	11	
Cmax (µg/ml)	0.89 (0.37)	1.42 (0.75)	0.015
Tmax (h)	1.0 (1.0-3.0)	2.0 (1.0-4.0)	ns
$T_{1/2}$ (h)	98 (64)	91 (33)	ns
AUC (µg•h/ml)	3.6 (1.7)	8.3 (3.2)	0.001

Data are means (± S.D.), except for Tmax, which is the median value and lower and upper range. Data are from Shah et al., 1992.

mechanism of action or in the occurrence of adverse effects in patients treated with ticlopidine.

Ticlopidine is extensively metabolized by the liver, and approximately 60% of an oral dose is excreted in urine.[10-12] Numerous metabolites of ticlopidine are present, but only trace levels of unmetabolized ticlopidine are detected (Figure 3.2). Most metabolites in urine result from metabolism of ticlopidine in the thiophene ring. In addition, approximately 6–15% of a dose of ticlopidine is metabolized to form o-chlorobenzoic acid, which is conjugated with glycine and excreted as o-chlorohippuric acid.

Pharmacokinetics in Healthy Subjects

Incidence of thromboembolic disease increases with age, and in general, the intended patient population for ticlopidine is elderly. For example, data which characterize ticlopidine's efficacy and safety for prevention of primary and recurrent stroke are based on large clinical trials in which the average age of subjects was 63 years[16] and 66 years.[17] Because clearance of many drugs decreases with increasing age, ticlopidine's pharmacokinetics after a single and multiple dose were compared in the young (mean age 29 years) and the elderly (mean age 70 years).[14] Indeed, plasma levels of ticlopidine are significantly higher and metabolic clearance of ticlopidine is significantly lower in elderly subjects as compared to young subjects (Table 3.1). As a result of this finding, subsequent pharmacokinetic and pharmacodynamic studies of ticlopidine were

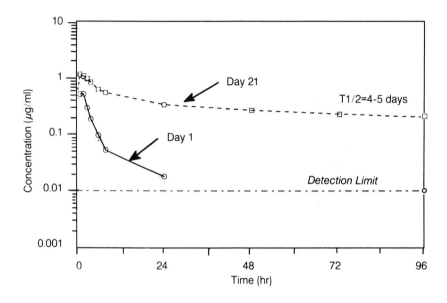

FIGURE 3.3. Concentrations of ticlopidine after a single 250 mg dose or after the last dose following multiple dosing with 250 mg bid for 21 days. Data represent the mean concentrations of ticlopidine in 11–12 subjects with an average age of 70 years.

performed in subjects closely approximating the intended patient population age for ticlopidine.

After administration of a single 250 mg dose of ticlopidine to elderly subjects, maximal concentrations (Cmax) in plasma occur approximately 2 hours after dosing (Tmax) and average 0.70 µg/ml (Table 3.1). After multiple dosing at 250 mg bid, steady-state trough levels are reached after approximately 14 days. In comparison to parameters obtained after a single dose, the value for Tmax is similar but Cmax is higher, averaging 1.4 µg/ml. After chronic dosing, measurable levels persist in plasma for several days after the last dose, and the half-life after multiple dosing averages 3.8 days (Figure 3.3). Substantially shorter half-lives of ticlopidine have been observed after single doses,[10,14,18] but these values are likely underestimates because of rapid decline of ticlopidine concentration in plasma to undetectable levels and the resultant failure to characterize the true elimination phase. In both young and elderly subjects given multiple doses of ticlopidine, values for AUC increase two to three times those observed after a single dose. This increase in AUC after multiple dosing is consistent with the threefold increase in [^{14}C]-ticlopidine described above[12] and may result from saturation of metabolism.

Pharmacodynamics

In Vitro Activity

At concentrations that occur in plasma after therapeutic doses, ticlopidine is essentially inactive as a platelet aggregation inhibitor when added directly to platelets. Only when substantially higher levels (300 μg/ml or greater) are added to platelet suspensions are ticlopidine's effects on platelet aggregation observed.[19] These concentrations are greater than 100 times the maximal levels of ticlopidine that circulate in plasma following therapeutic doses and probably result from nonspecific detergent effects of ticlopidine on the platelet membrane. Effects of very high concentrations on other pathways of platelet aggregation have been described (see reference 1 for review), but these observations are of doubtful relevance to the platelet effects observed following treatment with ticlopidine *in vivo*.

In Vivo Effects on Platelet Function

Template bleeding time,[20] which involves elevation of venous pressure with a cuff and determining bleeding duration from a small skin incision, is a simple and useful indicator of platelet function *in vivo*. Treatment with ticlopidine causes a time- and dose-dependent prolongation of bleeding time, but this effect is quite variable. As much as a fivefold increase in bleeding time is observed,[21] however, substantially less prolongation is observed when bleeding time is measured without elevation of venous blood pressure.[22] Bleeding times return to baseline values within 5–7 days after ticlopidine treatment is discontinued.[10]

Ex Vivo Effects on Platelet Function

Numerous pharmacodynamic studies of ticlopidine have been performed in healthy, young volunteers in which ticlopidine's effects on ADP-induced platelet aggregation were determined.[21-26] Inhibition of platelet function develops after multiple doses of ticlopidine, and the rate of onset and extent of inhibition is dose dependent. At a dose of 500 mg/day, significant inhibition of ADP-induced platelet aggregation is observed after 1–2 days, and full inhibition is obtained after 5–8 days. Sensitivity of platelets to exogenous ADP is reduced by ticlopidine treatment. As compared to platelets from control subjects, higher concentrations of ADP are required to produce a given aggregation response. In patients treated for as long as 1–3 years, inhibition of ADP-induced platelet aggregation is sustained throughout treatment period.[27,28] Approximately 1–2 weeks are required for platelet function to return to baseline values after discontinuation of treatment.

A recent multicenter double-blind, dose-ranging study provided a definitive characterization of ticlopidine's effects in elderly subjects (average age = 60 years). Platelet aggregation was measured in response to two concentrations of ADP, which were titrated for each subject before treatment with ticlopidine. The lower concentration represented the "threshold concentration," which was the lowest ADP concentration that initiated platelet aggregation, and the "high" concentration represented two times the threshold concentration. Onset of ADP-induced platelet aggregation inhibition and inhibition extent are dose-dependent, as illustrated by ticlopidine's effect on "high ADP"-induced platelet aggregation inhibition. The most rapid onset and highest levels of inhibition are observed for the 750 mg/day dose, which produces 50% inhibition after 4 days and reaches a near-maximal effect of 62.5% inhibition after 8 days of treatment. The 500 mg/day dose produces effects similar to that of the 750 mg/day dose, although the peak effect is not reached until 11 days after dosing. The lowest dose evaluated in this study, 125 mg/day, is clearly less effective than the three higher doses. At a dose of 500 mg/day, significant inhibition of ADP-induced platelet aggregation is observed for as long as 1 week after discontinuing ticlopidine (see Chapter 4, Figure 4.6).

Despite the apparent plateau of inhibitory activity within the range of 125 to 750 mg/day, trough concentrations of ticlopidine increase disproportionately greater than the increase in dose. With a twofold increase in dose from 125 mg bid to 250 mg bid, trough concentrations increase approximately threefold, and with an increase of one and a half in dose from 250 mg bid to 375 mg bid, trough concentrations on day 15 increased by approximately 1.9 times.

An alternate method of viewing dose response data for ticlopidine is to examine the proportion of subjects who respond to ticlopidine with given levels of platelet aggregation inhibition. At a given dose, the extent of ADP-induced platelet aggregation inhibition is variable from subject to subject. It is reasonable to expect that optimal clinical efficacy would be observed with doses resulting in a high proportion of subjects exhibiting a marked degree of platelet aggregation inhibition. At the 500 and 750 mg/day doses, consistently higher proportions of subjects attain higher levels of platelet aggregation inhibition as compared to the 125 and 250 mg/day doses.

Ticlopidine inhibits several biochemical responses that accompany platelet activation, such as release of platelet serotonin and ATP, and formation of malondialdehyde and thromboxane B_2.[1] By inhibiting platelet activation in response to ADP, ticlopidine inhibits activation of the platelet membrane glycoprotein (GPIIb/IIIa) to form the fibrinogen binding site.[26,29]

Relationship of ADP-Induced Platelet Aggregation Inhibition to Concentrations of Ticlopidine in Plasma

The data described above indicate that ticlopidine's concentration in plasma as well as its inhibitory effect on platelets escalate with increasing doses. As a result it should be apparent that across doses, increasing concentrations of ticlopidine in plasma correlate with increasing platelet aggregation inhibition. Correlation between platelet aggregation inhibition and ticlopidine concentration in plasma within subjects treated with the same dose is less apparent. *In vitro* studies indicate that ticlopidine in plasma does not directly inhibit platelet aggregation, and on this basis alone, a direct relationship between ticlopidine levels and platelet effects would not be anticipated. If metabolic activation is involved in ticlopidine activity, one might predict that low levels of ticlopidine in plasma may be associated with higher degrees of metabolic activation and platelet inhibition, but ticlopidine levels in plasma may be reflective of net metabolic clearance via both activation or inactivation pathways. The concentrations of ticlopidine in plasma and their effect on platelet aggregation are not temporally related. Peak concentrations after a single 250 mg dose occur within 2 hours after dosing, but 1–2 days of dosing are required before a significant effect on platelet aggregation is observed. On a temporal basis, platelet aggregation inhibition more closely parallels steady-state levels of ticlopidine in plasma. Both trough plasma levels and platelet aggregation inhibition require 10–14 days to reach maximal levels. After termination of dosing, ticlopidine's half-life is approximately 4 days, which is consistent with the 1- to 2-week period required for platelet function to return to baseline values.

Based on the above considerations, it is not surprising that a lack of correlation between platelet aggregation inhibition and ticlopidine concentration in plasma has been observed. In a study of the pharmacokinetics and pharmacodynamics of ticlopidine in normal subjects and in subjects with various thrombotic diseases, no correlation between plasma levels and platelet function was found.[30] Similarly, in the multicenter dose-ranging study in elderly patients described above, no correlation between trough plasma levels and platelet function was observed within the 125, 500 and 750 mg/day groups. However, for the 250 mg/day group, a weak although statistically significant inverse correlation was consistently observed. Perhaps elucidation and quantitation of a metabolic pathway which results in formation of the proximate active metabolite will strengthen the pharmacokinetic-pharmacodynamic relationship for ticlopidine.

Relationship of Platelet Aggregation Inhibition to Therapeutic Efficacy of Ticlopidine

While it may be anticipated that the therapeutic outcome of antiplatelet therapy is a direct function of the extent to which platelet aggregation is inhibited, this relationship has not been extensively evaluated in clinical trials of antithrombotic agents. Although it is possible to relate ticlopidine dose to an average platelet aggregation inhibition in a group of subjects, or even to the extent of platelet aggregation inhibition in an individual subject, little quantitative data exists to define the relationship between extent of inhibition and therapeutic efficacy in preventing or reducing incidence of thromboembolic disease. Defining this relationship may augment antithrombotic therapy success in that therapy could be adjusted to provide optimal antiplatelet effects. While the quantitative relationship of ADP-induced platelet aggregation inhibition to ticlopidine's therapeutic activity in preventing thrombotic disease is not known, this question was addressed in a trial to evaluate ticlopidine's effectiveness in preventing progression of nonproliferative retinopathy in diabetic patients (TIMAD Study Group, 1990).

Reduction in progression of retinal capillary aneurysms in these patients is directly correlated to extent of ADP-induced platelet aggregation inhibition. Patients treated with ticlopidine who exhibited 50% or greater inhibition of ADP-induced platelet aggregation demonstrated a marked reduction or even a reversal in rate of microaneurysm progression as compared to patients on placebo or those on ticlopidine with less than 50% inhibition of ADP-induced platelet aggregation. Although diabetic retinopathy is caused by microaneurysms and is not a thrombotic dis- ease, results of this trial suggest that defining the relationship between inhibi- tion of platelet aggregation and therapeutic effectiveness in thromboembolic diseases will contribute to the effective use of ticlopidine and other antiplatelet agents.

Pharmacodynamics and Pharmacokinetics in Special Populations

Ticlopidine's pharmacodynamic effects have been determined in several diseases for which ticlopidine has been evaluated for therapeutic efficacy, such as patients with ischemic heart disease, cerebrovascular disease, diabetes and peripheral vascular disease.[1] Most studies have not utilized healthy volunteers as controls. In general it appears that the pharmacodynamic effects of ticlopidine in these studies are similar to those observed in studies of healthy volunteers, and pharmacokinetic differences between these patients and healthy age-matched volunteers are not anticipated. A reduced effect of ticlopidine on bleeding time and ADP-induced platelet aggregation in myocardial infarction patients in comparison to healthy volunteers has been reported.[31]

Ticlopidine inhibits several parameters of platelet function in patients with renal disease. Although ticlopidine is cleared almost entirely by metabolism, studies in subjects with varying degrees of renal function demonstrate that there is a trend toward higher concentrations of ticlopidine with decreasing renal function. Other than a somewhat greater prolongation of cuffed bleeding time in patients with moderate impairment of renal function as compared to normals, ticlopidine treatment is well tolerated and results in similar inhibition of ADP-induced platelet aggregation in normal subjects and subjects with mild or moderate impairment of renal function.

Caution should be used in treatment of patients with hepatic disease and its associated coagulation disorders since ticlopidine significantly inhibits platelet function. A study in which patients with hepatic cirrhosis were given ticlopidine at a dose of 250 mg bid for 15 days or longer indicated that ticlopidine concentrations in plasma may be elevated in patients with hepatic disease. Ticlopidine's effect on ADP-induced platelet aggregation was somewhat reduced in these patients, although it was well tolerated and did not affect coagulation parameters.

Drug Interactions

There are several studies examining potential interactions with co-administered drugs. Therapeutic doses of ticlopidine cause a 30% increase in plasma half-life of antipyrine,[32] a model compound that is eliminated almost entirely by hepatic metabolism. Thus ticlopidine may cause a modest reduction in clearance of similarly metabolized drugs. Consistent with this prediction, it was reported that concomitant administration of ticlopidine increases elimination half-life of theophylline from 8.6 to 12.2 hours and produces a comparable reduction in total plasma clearance of theophylline.[33] Drugs that themselves reduce hepatic drug metabolism may reduce metabolism of ticlopidine, as evident by the finding that chronic administration of cimetidine reduces clearance of a single dose of ticlopidine by approximately 50%. The pharmacodynamic consequence of this interaction is unknown but is currently under investigation. Administration of ticlopidine after antacids results in a small (20%) decrease in plasma AUC for ticlopidine.[18]

Co-administration of ticlopidine with digoxin did not alter peak or trough levels but resulted in a slight decrease (approximately 15%) in the plasma AUC for digoxin.[34] Binding of ticlopidine to plasma protein was not affected by therapeutic concentrations of propranolol or phenytoin. Likewise, binding of propranolol and phenytoin to plasma proteins was not affected by ticlopidine.

Pharmacodynamic interactions with respect to platelet aggregation inhibition have been characterized for the combination of ticlopidine with aspirin.[22] Ticlopidine (250 mg bid for 5 days) inhibits the primary phase of ADP- induced platelet aggregation but aspirin (550 mg tid for 5 days) does not. Both ticlopidine and aspirin inhibit collagen-induced aggregation, although the effect of aspirin is stronger. Simultaneous administration of aspirin with ticlopidine does not modify the ticlopidine-mediated inhibition of ADP-induced platelet aggregation, but ticlopidine potentiates aspirin's effect on collagen-induced platelet aggregation. Use of this combination in prevention of thromboembolic disease has not been extensively evaluated.

Administration of corticosteroids reverses ticlopidine-induced prolongation of bleeding time but does not alter ticlopidine-mediated inhibition of ADP-induced platelet aggregation.[35] Treatment with corticosteroids has been suggested as a method for controlling excessive bleeding caused by ticlopidine.[35]

References

1. Saltiel E, Ward A. Ticlopidine, a review of its pharmacodynamic and pharmacokinetic properties, and therapeutic efficacy in platelet-dependent disease states. *Drugs* 1987; **34**:222–262.
2. Fèliste R, Delebassée D, Simon MF, Chap H, Defeyn G, Vallée E, Douste-Blazy L, Maffrand JP. Broad spectrum anti-platelet activity of ticlopidine and PCR 4099 involves the suppression of the effects of released ADP. *Thromb Res* 1987;**48**;403–415.
3. Born GVR. Aggregation of blood platelets by adenosine diphosphate and its reversal. *Nature* 1962;**194**:927–929.
4. Bruno JJ. The mechanisms of action of ticlopidine. *Thromb Res* 1983;Suppl 4:59–67.
5. di Minno G, Cerbone AM, Mattioli PL, Turco S, Iovine C, Mancini M. Functionally thrombasthenic state in normal platelets following the administration of ticlopidine. *J Clin Invest* 1985;**75**:328–338.
6. Aubert D, Bernat A, Ferrand J, Maffrand JP, Szygenda E, et al. Pharmacological profile of PCR 3787: a metabolite of ticlopidine. Seventh International Congress of Thrombosis, 1982.
7. Vincent JE, Zijlstra FJ, de Wit CM, Bonta IL. The effect of 5-(2-chlorobenzyl)-5,6,7,7a-tetrahydro 4H-thieno (3,2-c)-pyridine-2-one hydrochloride (PCR 3787), a metabolite of ticlopidine, on the aggregation of human platelets *in vitro* and on the aggregation action of PGI$_2$ and PGD$_2$. *Prost Leukotri Med* 1984;**16**:279–283.
8. McTavish D, Faulds D, Goa KL. Ticlopidine: an updated review of its pharmacology and therapeutic use in platelet dependent disorders. *Drugs* 1990;**40**:238–259.
9. Bruno JJ, Malony BA. Ticlopidine. *New Drugs Annual: Cardiovascular Drugs* 1983;295–316.
10. Panak EA, Maffrand JP, Picard-Fraire C, Vallée E, Blanchard JF, Roncucci R. Ticlopidine: a promise for the prevention and treatment of thrombosis and its complications. *Hæmostasis* 1983;**13**(suppl 1):154.
11. Picard-Fraire C. Pharmacokinetic and metabolic characteristics of ticlopidine in relation to its inhibitory properties on platelet function. *Agents and Actions Suppl* 1984;**15**:68–75.
12. Teitelbaum P, Gabuzda TG, Koretz SH, Massey I, Molony B. Pharmacokinetics of ticlopidine in young and old adult subjects following single and multiple dosing (abstract). *J Pharmaceut Sci* 1987;**76**:599.
13. Syntex Research. Unpublished data on file.
14. Shah J, Teitelbaum P, Molony BA, Gabuzda T, Massey I. Single and multiple dose pharmacokinetics of ticlopidine in young and elderly subjects. *Br J Pharmacol* (in press).
15. Glasson S, Zini R, Tillement JP. Multiple human serum binding of two thienopyridinic derivatives, ticlopidine and PCR 2362, and their distribution between HSA, α_1-acid glycoprotein and lipoproteins. *Biochem Pharmacol* 1982;**31**:831–835.

16. Hass WK, Easton JD, Adams HP, Pryse-Philips W, Molony BA, Anderson S, Kamm B. A randomized trial comparing ticlopidine hydrochloride with aspirin for the prevention of stroke in high-risk patients. *N Engl J Med* 1989;**321**:501–507.

17. Gent M, Easton JD, Hachinski VC, Panak EA, Sicurella J, Blakely JA, Ellis DL, et al. The Canadian American Ticlopidine Study (CATS) in Thromboembolic Stroke. *Lancet* 1989;**1**:1215–1220.

18. Shah J, Fratis A, Ellis D, Murakami S, Teitelbaum P. Effect of food and antacid on absorption of orally administered ticlopidine hydrochloride. *J Clin Pharmacol* 1990;**30**: 733–736.

19. Bruno JJ, Yang D, Taylor LA, Feamster C. Role of platelet cAMP and prostacyclin synthesis in platelet aggregation inhibition by ticlopidine hydrochloride (abstract). *Thromb Haemost* 1981;**46**:66.

20. Mielke CH, Kaneshira MM, Weiner JM, Rapaport SI. The standardized normal Ivy bleeding time and its prolongation by aspirin. *Blood* 1960;**34**:204–215.

21. David JL, Monfort F, Herion F, Raskinet R. Compared effects of three dose-levels of ticlopidine on platelet function in normal subjects. *Thromb Res* 1979;**14**:35–49.

22. Thebault JJ, Blatrix CE, Blanchard JF, Panak EA. The interactions of ticlopidine and aspirin in normal subjects. *J Int Med Res* 1977;**5**:405–411.

23. Thebault JJ, Blatrix CE, Blanchard JF, Panak EA. Effects of ticlopidine, a new platelet aggregation inhibitor in man. *Clin Pharmacol Therapeutics* 1975;**18**:485–490.

24. Ellis DL, Roe RL, Bruno JJ, Cranston BJ, McSpadden MM. The effects of ticlopidine hydrochloride on bleeding time and platelet function in man (abstract). *Thromb Haemost* 1981;**46**:176.

25. Bruno JJ, Chang L, McSpadden M, Yang D. The effect of oral ticlopidine on arachidonic acid products in human platelets. *Agents and Actions Suppl* 1984;**15**:76–87.

26. Iovine C, d'Avenia V, Turco S, Mattioli P, di Minno G. *Ex vivo* effects of ticlopidine on human platelets: inhibition of fibrinogen binding by a mechanism independent of thromboxane formation. *Agents and Actions Suppl* 1984;**15**:105–107.

27. Conrad J, LeCrubier C, Scarabin PY, Horellow MH, Samama M, Bousser MG. Effects of long term administration of ticlopidine on platelet function and hemostatic variables. *Thromb Res* 1980;**20**:143–148.

28. Mirouze J, et al. (TIMAD Study Group). Ticlopidine treatment reduces the progression of non-proliferative diabetic retinopathy. *Arch Opthalmol* 1990;**108**:1577–1583.

29. Dunn F, Soria J, Soria C, Thomaidis A, Lee H, et al. *In vivo* effect of ticlopidine on fibrinogen-platelet cofactor activity and binding of fibrinogen to platelets. *Agents and Actions Suppl* 1984;**15**:97–104.

30. Knudsen JB, Gormsen J. The effect of ticlopidine on platelet function in normal volunteers and in patients with platelet hyperaggregability *in vitro*. *Thromb Res* 1979; **16**:663–671.

31. Meschengieser S, Woods A, Schattner M, Lazzari M. Antiplatelet action of ticlopidine on normal patients and thrombotic patients (abstract). Seventh International Congress on Thrombosis, 1982, p 159.

32. Thebault JJ, Blatrix CE, Blanchard JF, Panak EA. Effect of ticlopidine treatment on liver metabolizing enzymes in man. *Br J Clin Pharmacol* 1980;**10**:311–313.

33. Colli A, Buccino G, Cocciolo M, Parravicini R, Elli GM, Scaltrini G. Ticlopidine— theophylline interaction. *Clin Pharmacol Ther* 1987;**41**:358362.

34. Vargas R, Reitman M, Teitelbaum P, Ryan JR, McMahon FG, Jain AK, Ryan M, Regel
    G. Study of the effect of ticlopidine on digoxin blood levels (Abstract). *Clin Pharmacol
    Ther* 1988;**43**:176.
35. Thebault JJ, Blatrix CE, Blanchard JF, Panak EA. A possible method to control
    prolongations of bleeding time under antiplatelet therapy with ticlopidine. *Thromb
    Haemost* 1982;**48**:6–8.

4
Ticlopidine's Mechanism of Action on Human Platelets

LAURENCE A. HARKER and JOHN J. BRUNO

Rationale for the Clinical Use of Platelet Aggregation Inhibiting Agents

Platelets and Thrombosis

The importance of platelets in thromboembolic disease has been documented in studies over the past three decades. Morphologic studies in patients who died of cardiovascular and cerebrovascular disease have shown the presence of platelets in both venous and arterial thrombi. Thrombus formation is influenced by the rheologic properties of blood in the vasculature in which they are formed. Thus, thrombi formed in venous and arterial systems differ in composition. Thrombi formed in the venous system, where blood flow is slow and stasis often exists, are composed of fibrin and blood cells in the approximate proportion in which they are found in whole blood. In the arterial system, where blood flow is rapid and nonlaminar and where higher shear conditions prevail, thrombi formed are composed chiefly of platelets and, to a variable degree, fibrin and other blood cells, depending to some extent on thrombus age and conditions under which it is formed.[1] Thrombosis and atherosclerosis are intimately and closely involved in coronary artery disease, peripheral vascular disease, and cerebrovascular disease. In addition, closure of vascular grafts after coronary artery bypass surgery and the restenosis seen after coronary and peripheral angioplasty are known to have a significant platelet involvement.[2] Furthermore, in patients who died from "sudden cardiac death," autopsy performed within 35 hours of death revealed platelet microthrombi in the intramyocardial vasculature more frequently than in the intramyocardial vasculature of patients who died from noncardiovascular causes.[3]

Platelets and Hemostasis

Hemostasis, the process by which loss of blood from acute breaks in blood vessels is staunched, has three main components: 1) vascular vasomotor mechanisms; 2) cellular constituents of blood, which are primarily related to platelet

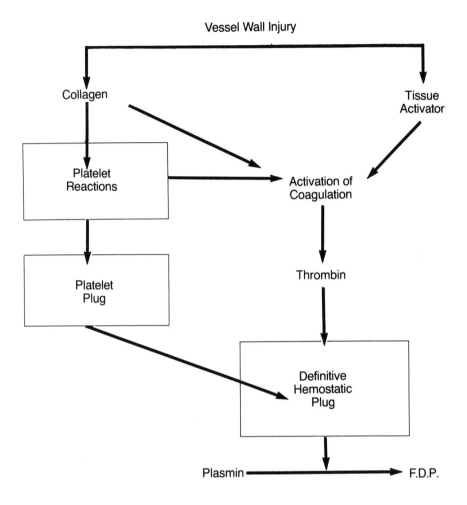

FIGURE 4.1. The hemostatic apparatus. Simplified outline of hemostatic pathway indicating interaction between the soluble components of hemostasis (activation of coagulation) and the cellular (platelet reactions) component.

accumulation; and 3) soluble plasma proteins, constituting the coagulation and fibrinolytic cascades. There are important multiple and complex interactions among components of the vessel wall, platelets and other blood cells, serine proteases comprising the coagulation and fibrinolytic pathways, and the many mechanisms in blood and blood vessels regulating these processes (Figure 4.1).

Platelets are the smallest formed elements in blood. These anucleate blood cells have many of the subcellular organelles associated with nucleated cells,

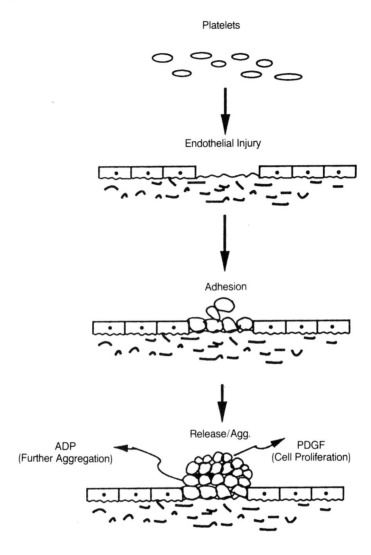

FIGURE 4.2. Schematic diagram of platelet response to injury of a blood vessel. In the final stage, platelets begin to aggregate and release ADP which induces aggregation of nearby platelets. The platelets release PDGF which is rapidly taken up by smooth muscle cells (SMC) and which induces proliferation of the SMC.

including mitochondria, various granules with secretory function, and contractile proteins that control both platelet shape and secretion of granule contents. Platelets are important in the hemostatic apparatus. In the absence of injury, platelets circulate as discoid bodies and contribute to maintenance of vascular integrity by sealing over any minor breaks. After vascular injury, platelets are activated by various stimuli, including ADP and thrombin, or by contact with collagen or other subendothelial connective tissue matrix material. They adhere at the injury site and release granular material, whereby they recruit other platelets and form aggregates. This mass of platelets forms the initial hemostatic plug.

Formation of a thrombus involves similar processes. Under pathologic conditions vascular injury may be produced by chemical, immunological, or physical factors, or may follow rupture of a stenotic atherosclerotic lesion in the coronary or cerebral vasculature, leading to thrombo-occlusion and consequent heart attack or stroke (Figure 4.2).

Platelet Aggregation Inhibiting Drugs in Clinical Trials

Development of antiplatelet agents for treatment of patients with vascular disease has been a scientifically complex and slow process.[4] When evaluation of ticlopidine was initiated in the United States in 1979, several platelet aggregation inhibitory drugs had been studied in clinical trials to prevent thromboembolic events. Aspirin was studied in a large multicenter clinical trial, the Aspirin Myocardial Infarction Study (AMIS), for prevention of nonfatal and fatal secondary myocardial infarction (MI) and death.[5] Aspirin, together with dypyridamole, was also examined in a study similar to AMIS, the Persantine Aspirin Reinfarction Study (PARIS), for prevention of the same events,[6] and sulfinpyrazone was studied in the Anturane Reinfarction Trial (ART) to prevent myocardial deaths.[7] Although none of these trials achieved acceptable statistical significance, both studies involving aspirin displayed trends toward prevention of reinfarction and death.

In the late 1970s, a clinical trial for prevention of threatened stroke, the Canadian Cooperative Study,[8] was successfully completed. This study had four groups: aspirin, sulfinpyrazone, a combination of the two, and a placebo group. Sulfinpyrazone alone was no different from placebo. The two treatment groups with aspirin alone and in combination with sulfinpyrazone had identical strong trends toward reducing nonfatal and fatal stroke. When both the aspirin groups were combined, a statistically significant reduction of nonfatal and fatal stroke in males was seen. On the basis of this study, aspirin received FDA approval for use in prevention of threatened stroke in males.

Subsequently, in a Veterans Administration-sponsored study of men with preinfarction angina, aspirin was shown to be successful in reducing acute myocardial infarction (MI) and death in patients with unstable angina.[9] On the basis of a subsequent meta-analysis of all aspirin studies of secondary prevention of MI (involving 18,000 patients), aspirin was determined to be useful in prevention of nonfatal and fatal MI.[10] Aspirin is now recommended for prevention of both threatened and recurrent MI.

Rationale for the Study of Ticlopidine in Thromboembolic Disease

There were two important reasons for selecting ticlopidine as the intervention in clinical trials evaluating thromboembolic events: first, ticlopidine is a global inhibitor of platelet recruitment; second, ticlopidine activity is permanent for the platelet's lifetime.

Studies of the mechanisms mediating platelet activation indicate that there are at least three important and interrelated pathways leading to platelet recruitment: 1) ADP released from erythrocytes or secreted from storage (dense) granules of stimulated platelets; 2) subendothelial connective tissue constituents, primarily collagen; and 3) thrombin.[1]

It was shown that ADP released from erythrocytes causes platelets to aggregate.[11] *In vitro* whole blood bleeding time studies demonstrated that enzymes destroying ADP prolong bleeding times.[12] It was subsequently demonstrated in animal experiments that ADP-utilizing enzymes prolong time required for platelets to form hemostatic plugs.[13] Furthermore, it was also shown that ADP initiates platelet thrombus formation *in vivo* by microiontophoretic injection of ADP into the vasculature; thrombi form at the site of iontophoresis.[14]

ADP, collagen, and thrombin initiate fibrinogen binding site expression on platelet membranes by inducing a conformational change in the GPIIb/IIIa complex, the final common pathway of platelet aggregation/recruitment.[15] Absence of GPIIb/IIIa or inability to stimulate expression of the fibrinogen binding site results in a markedly prolonged bleeding time.[16,17] Aspirin, the only other agent approved for reduction of thromboembolic events in patients with vascular disease, induces irreversible inactivation of platelet cyclooxygenase. Aspirin does not inhibit primary ADP-induced aggregation or ADP-induced exposure of the platelet fibrinogen receptor. Bleeding time prolongation after aspirin ingestion is similar to that seen in patients having defects in enzymes of the cyclooxygenase system and results in only mild prolongation of bleeding time measurements.[18]

Although most nonsteroidal antiinflammatory drugs (NSAIDS) inhibit platelet production of thromboxane synthesized by the cyclooxygenase system, aspirin is the only one that does this irreversibly. No doubt this property of aspirin contributes to its usefulness as an antiplatelet agent and distinguishes aspirin from other NSAIDS.

Ticlopidine resembles aspirin in that it irreversibly inhibits expression of the GPIIb/IIIa receptor for fibrinogen binding after oral administration, thereby decreasing platelet aggregation/recruitment and causing prolongation of bleeding time measurements. However, ticlopidine differs from aspirin in that it also inhibits the two more powerful platelet agonists, collagen and thrombin, and it is ineffective *in vitro*, requiring several days of oral administration before achieving its full antiplatelet capacity.

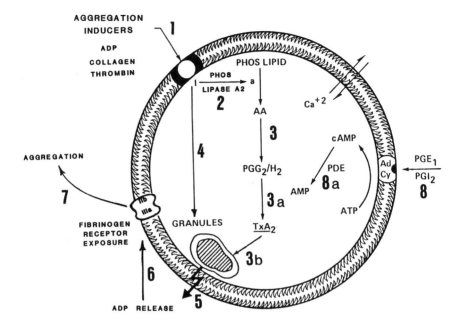

FIGURE 4.3. Schematic diagram showing important pathways of platelet aggregation and inhibition. Inducers acting at specific receptors (generically shown, Step 1) stimulate release of ADP from platelet dense granules (Step 5) via arachidonic acid release and synthesis of thromboxane A_2 (Step 3–3b), or by direct action (Step 4), leading to exposure of the fibrinogen receptor, GPIIb/IIIa (Step 6), and platelet aggregation (Step 7). Aggregation inhibitors can antagonize inducers (Steps 1, 3b), prevent granule release (Step 4), elevate intraplatelet cAMP (Steps 8, 8a) and thus prevent platelet activation by most inducers. Aspirin inhibits the synthesis of all cyclooxygenase products (Step 3), including thromboxane A_2, and thus, its subsequent action. Ticlopidine is believed to inhibit the transduction of signal from inducers (Step 6), e.g., ADP, and thus prevent exposure of fibrinogen receptors and platelet aggregation.

Ticlopidine's Mode of Action

Introduction

Ticlopidine is an antiplatelet agent with a unique mechanism of action different from the presently known agents, including aspirin, the only FDA approved, platelet-inhibiting drug now available for prevention of stroke, MI, or vascular death. Ticlopidine acts by inhibiting all three pathways of platelet activation. At the currently used clinical dosage, inhibitory effects are most readily demonstrated using ADP as the agonist, although other pathways by which antiplatelet agents act will also be discussed. In addition, ticlopidine acts irreversibly on

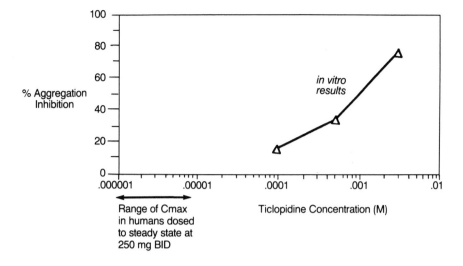

FIGURE 4.4. Inhibition of platelet aggregation by ticlopidine added to platelet-rich plasma in vitro.

platelets, a characteristic that maintains inhibition of platelet function despite an occasional missed dose. A comparison of ticlopidine with available known platelet-inhibiting drugs demonstrates that ticlopidine has properties suggesting that it may have advantages over other available agents.

Ticlopidine is a platelet aggregation inhibitor that is structurally different from other known antithrombotic agents and that has a mechanism of action not yet elucidated. Many studies have been performed in an attempt to understand ticlopidine's mechanism of action; however, the molecular mechanism is still not known.

All agonists of platelet aggregation act at platelet receptors specific for the particular agonist (Figure 4.3), inducing a chain of events giving rise to signal transduction. The result is formation of platelet aggregates *in vitro* and thrombi *in vivo*. In the ticlopidine studies to be presented, ADP is the agonist generally used. It acts at a platelet membrane receptor not yet fully characterized (Figure 4.3, Step 1).

In Vitro Studies

Customarily, platelet aggregation inhibitors are studied by adding the potential inhibitor to a suspension of platelet rich in plasma (PRP) obtained by centrifugation of whole blood. Addition of an inducer to the PRP, containing the putative inhibitor, leads to varying degrees of aggregation. The results are compared with aggregation in PRP alone to determine the inhibition caused by the agent added.

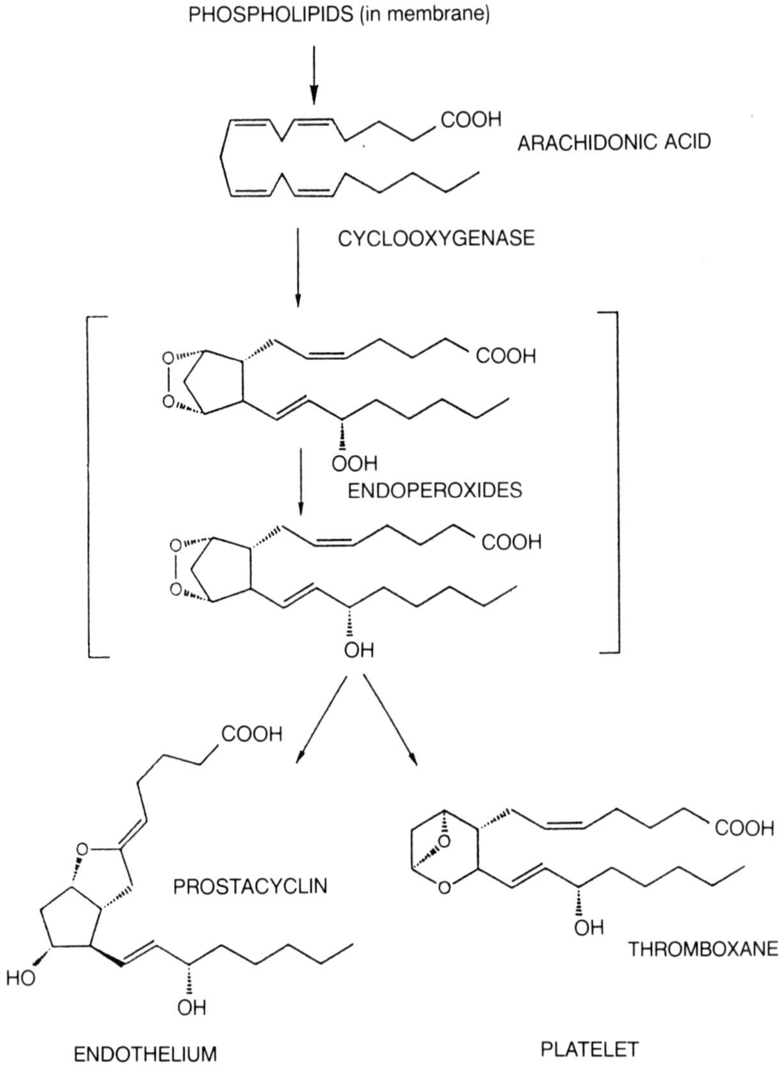

FIGURE 4.5. Percent inhibition of ADP-induced platelet aggregation by days in a study of 116 subjects of 50–75 years of age. The subjects were dosed as indicated for 14 days. For the two higher doses, maximum inhibition is achieved after 8–11 days of treatment. Both the onset and offset of inhibition are shown to be dose-dependent.

When ticlopidine is added *in vitro* to PRP, it fails to inhibit platelet aggregation significantly, regardless of which species' PRP is used. Concentrations required for aggregation inhibition *in vitro* are many orders of magnitude higher than the peak plasma levels found *in vivo*. When ticlopidine is studied in the PRP of rats, rabbits, and humans, IC_{50} values for aggregation inhibition induced by ADP are 1 μM, whereas peak plasma concentrations of ticlopidine, which exhibit maximum *ex vivo* inhibition of platelet aggregation, are in the range of 1 to 5 μM (Figure 4.4) after therapeutic doses (250 mg bid) to volunteers.[19] Similar plasma levels were found in animals.[20]

Ex Vivo Studies

Ex vivo aggregation studies are carried out in the same manner as described above except that the drug is administered orally to an animal or human before the blood sample is taken. When ticlopidine is administered orally, there is a time- and dose-dependent onset of inhibition of ADP-induced platelet aggregation. A multicenter dose-ranging study illustrating these points was recently completed in a population of subjects (N = 116) of the same age as patients in the Canadian American Ticlopidine Study (CATS)[21] (Figure 4.5). As in other studies, time to onset of activity and extent of inhibition are dose related. For the 500 mg/day regimen, peak effect is seen 8–11 days after dosing begins. Onset of activity is somewhat faster for the 750 mg/day dose, but maximum inhibition of platelet aggregation is similar by day 15.

When dosing is stopped, there is a time-dependent offset of platelet aggregation inhibiting activity that is consistent with an irreversible platelet alteration, as in the case of irreversible inhibition of the platelet cyclooxygenase by aspirin. The duration of this offset effect for ticlopidine parallels the half-life of a human platelet. A similar effect is observed in the rat.[22]

Comparison of Ticlopidine with Other Platelet Aggregation Inhibitors

Comparison was made of the effects of ticlopidine, aspirin, aspirin plus dipyridamole, and sulfinpyrazole on several platelet functions (Table 4.1). The 12 subjects in this crossover study (ICM 830) were dosed for 4 days according to the regimen shown in Table 4.2, which also presents comparison results. Note that ticlopidine is the only agent that significantly inhibits all the indices of platelet function.

Subjects in this study were dosed with ticlopidine for only 4 days. It is probable that had dosing continued for 8–11 days, i.e., to maximum aggregation inhibiting potential, inhibition of platelet retention on glass beads would have been even greater. Inhibition of platelet retention on glass beads has been shown to be a function of ADP released, either from platelets or more likely from erythrocytes.[11] It is possible that ticlopidine inhibits platelet retention on glass beads

TABLE 4.1. Comparison of ticlopidine, aspirin, aspirin plus dipyridamole, and sulfin-pyrazone on indices of platelet function (ICM 830).

Drug regimen	ADP-induced aggregation % inhibition	Epinephrine-induced aggregation % inhibition	Retention of glass beads % inhibition	Bleeding time % increase
Aspirin 650 mg bid	0	84[1]	4.5	83[1]
Aspirin 650 mg bid + dipyridamole 50 mg tid	20[1]	68[1]	2.5	117[1]
Sulfinpyrazone 200 mg qid	14[1]	41[1]	1.3	26[1]
Ticlopidine 250 mg bid	64[1]	63[1]	17.5[1]	161[1]

[1] p < 0.05 for one sample t-test (within group) on difference from 0 hour or day 1.

because it alone of the agents tested inhibits ADP-induced platelet activation. However, other possibilities have not been eliminated.

Involvement of Metabolites

Observations of ticlopidine—that it is essentially inactive when added directly to PRP, that oral administration results in inhibitory activity, and that this inhibition is irreversible as implied by offset of activity data—suggest that ticlopidine depends on metabolic processing to be active and that this metabolism permanently alters the platelet.

Since it was reported that a circulating metabolite in the plasma of ticlopi-dine-treated subjects inhibited aggregation of platelets from untreated individuals,[23] experiments have been carried out to investigate this possibility.

When platelets from untreated individuals were resuspended in plasma from subjects dosed for 7 days with ticlopidine, no inhibition of platelet aggregation was observed (Table 4.3), indicating that circulating, stable metabolites of ticlopidine do not directly inhibit platelet aggregation. When platelets from treated individuals were resuspended in plasma from either group, inhibition of ADP-induced aggregation was found. Inhibition of platelet aggregation apparently is not mediated by stable, circulating metabolites in plasma. This study clearly shows that ticlopidine's effect is permanently associated with the platelet.

The only identified metabolite of ticlopidine that exhibits antiplatelet effects is 2-hydroxy ticlopidine (2-HT). It significantly inhibits platelet aggregation, but similar to ticlopidine, it requires oral administration to exhibit its full antiplatelet effects. Like ticlopidine, 2-HT is inactive *in vitro* and has not been detected (< 0.05 g/ml) in plasma of rats, mice, rhesus monkeys, baboons, or humans given oral doses of ticlopidine. Production of ticlopidine to 2-HT may represent an initial metabolic step that results in formation of an active metabolite.

Although ticlopidine's effects on platelet inhibition of agents that stimulate or inhibit drug metabolism have been examined in several studies, results of these studies are equivocal.[19,20,22] Thus, the role of metabolized ticlopidine in

TABLE 4.2. Prolongation of bleeding time after ticlopidine treatment. (ICM-1369) bleeding time and aggregation study).

		Bleeding time (min)		
	Subject	Pre	Post	Aggregation inhibition (%)
2 hours postdose	1	3.00	14.00	1.50*
	4	5.50	20.50	69.00
	6	4.50	24.50	70.00
	9	5.50	32.00	72.00
	10	3.00	15.00	80.00
	12	6.00	33.00	89.00
	MEAN	4.58	23.17	63.58
12 hours postdose				76.00**
	2	4.50	67.50	67.00
	3	4.50	42.50	77.00
	5	5.50	11.50	74.00
	7	5.50	15.50	77.00
	8	2.50	60.00	89.00
	11	4.00	75.00	84.00
	MEAN	4.42	45.33	78.00
	OVERALL MEAN	4.51	33.40	70.65

*After wash, % inhibition was 70–80%.
**Mean omitting subject #1.

development of platelet aggregation inhibition remains unclear. Slow onset of activity and failure to find an active circulating metabolite have led to speculation that ticlopidine itself may act to inhibit platelets during megakaryocytopoiesis and subsequent platelet production in the bone marrow. However, there are no direct data to confirm this postulate.

Arachidonic Acid Metabolism

Induction of platelet aggregation by low to moderate concentrations of inducers activates two major pathways of aggregation in human platelets: that mediated byproducts of the arachidonic acid (AA) pathway (Figure 4.3, Steps 2, 3, 3a, 3b), and that initiated by direct release (Figure 4.3, Steps 4–5) of products from platelet-dense granules, especially ADP (Figure 4.3, Step 5). Activation of the AA pathway may be blocked by AA release inhibitors from the platelet membrane (Step 2) or at any point after AA release along the pathway from Step 3 to 3b (Figure 4.3). NSAIDS inhibit the cyclooxygenase enzyme (Figure 4.3, Step 3) that converts AA to endoperoxides, leading to immediate production of thromboxane A2 (T × A2). Aspirin, as noted, differs from other NSAIDS in that it irreversibly inhibits Step 3. It seems probable that the irreversible inhibition

TABLE 4.3. Reconstitution of platelets and platelet-poor plasma from ticlopidine-treated and control subjects' effect on ADP-induced platelet aggregation (ICM 1369 II).

Platlet	Plasma	N	Incubation time (min)	Aggregation (% transmittance)	% inhibition
Control	Control	9	0	68.5 ± 4.9	0
			30	64.0 ± 8.5	0
			90	44.0 ± 9.9	0
Treated	Treated		0	7.5 ± 5.7	89[1]
	Autologous	12	30	10.5 ± 5.4	84[1]
			90	9.1 ± 4.0	79[1]
Treated	Control	12	0	8.7 ± 5.2	87[1]
			30	10.3 ± 4.9	84[1]
			90	9.9 ± 4.0	78[1]
Control	Treated	12	0	62.3 ± 15.6	9
			30	58.6 ± 22.0	8
			90	53.0 ± 20.9	−20

[1] $p < 0.001$.

of cyclooxygenase confers an advantage for aspirin over other NSAIDS. Plasma levels of aspirin are irrelevant to its inhibition of the platelet enzyme, but this is not so for other, reversible inhibitors of cyclooxygenase, which may account for the finding that of all NSAIDS, only aspirin has been shown clinically to reduce the incidence of thromboembolic events.

Ticlopidine does not inhibit cyclooxygenase directly, although the secondary synthesis of TXA_2 by platelets may be inhibited by ticlopidine treatment because of its broad effects on platelet reactivity. Thromboxane production 6 minutes after collagen challenge of the PRP of volunteers, dosed for 7 days with ticlopidine (250 mg, bid), is inhibited 62% compared with pretreatment production (Table 4.4A). At the same time, platelet aggregation is inhibited 75%. There is also a trend toward inhibition of 12-HETE, the AA product of the platelet 12-lipoxygenase enzyme, although because of variability, this did not reach statistical significance.[24] When platelets of these same volunteers are washed and resuspended in buffer, TXA_2 made from exogenously added 14C-AA is not inhibited, even though collagen-induced platelet aggregation is 88% inhibited (Table 4.4B).[24] This result suggests that ticlopidine does not inhibit synthesis of the cyclooxygenase system.

Collagen activation of platelets stimulates release of platelet AA and synthesis of TXA_2, resulting in release of ADP from platelet-dense granules and platelet aggregation.[25] NSAIDS at high enough concentrations will completely inhibit TXA_2 formation and release of ADP from platelet granules. However, ticlopidine at higher doses inhibits platelet activation by collagen at collagen concentrations that overcome the effects of aspirin and other NSAIDS.[26] Thus, inhibition of collagen-induced platelet aggregation/recruitment by ticlopidine results from

TABLE 4.4. Effect of ticlopidine treatment on collagen-induced platelet aggregation and on platelet thromboxane production (ICM 1102).

Group	N	TXB_2, ng/10^9 platelets[1]	Percent inhibition	
			TXB_2 Synthesis	Collagen aggregation
A. *In human PRP*				
Predose	6	104 ± 74	0	0
Postdose[2]	6	33 ± 15	62 ± 20^3	75 ± 28^3
B. *In human washed resuspended platelets with 4 μM ^{14}C-AA added 3 minutes before collagen challenge*				
Predose	6	855 ± 81	NA	0
Postdose	6	869 ± 207	NA	88 ± 11^3

Entries are means ± standard deviation.

[1] TXB_2 was used as an indicator of TXA_2 concentrations, TXB_2 measurements were made 6 minutes after collagen addition.

[2] Seven days dosing with 250 mg bid; blood sample taken 12 hours after final dose.

[3] $p < .001$, paired t-test comparison with individual baseline data.

interruption of other mechanisms of activation than AA generation, thromboxane production, or ADP stimulation.

In this regard, ticlopidine has a theoretical advantage over aspirin. Aspirin inhibits production of prostacyclin (PGI2), a cyclooxygenase product of the vascular endothelium (Figure 4.6) and a powerful inhibitor of platelet activation (Figure 4.3, Step 8). PGI2 released from the vascular endothelium is postulated to be an *in vivo* regulator of thrombosis. Ticlopidine does not inhibit PGI2 synthesis.[27]

Platelet Cyclic AMP

Agents that elevate platelet cyclic AMP (cAMP), such as prostacyclin and cAMP phosphodiesterase (PDE) inhibitors (Figure 4.3, Steps 8 and 8a), prevent the rise in cytosolic Ca++ concentration leading to platelet activation. It was reported several years ago that inhibition of platelet function by ticlopidine may result from elevation of platelet cAMP after ticlopidine treatment.[28] The authors suggested that ticlopidine inhibited platelet cAMP PDE; however, direct measurements failed to show that ticlopidine inhibits cAMP PDE.[29]

Other investigators have confirmed that small but significant increases in intracellular cAMP occur in platelets from ticlopidine-treated animals and humans.[30,31] Recent studies demonstrate that ticlopidine treatment results in the selective suppression of ADP-mediated platelet adenylate cyclase inhibition.[32,33] Despite these reports other experiments cast doubt that cAMP plays any significant role in ticlopidine's mechanism of action. Agents that inhibit platelet aggregation by elevating cAMP have this inhibition reversed by 9-(tetrahydro-2-furyl) adenine (SQ-22536), an inhibitor of adenylate cyclase. SQ-22536, added

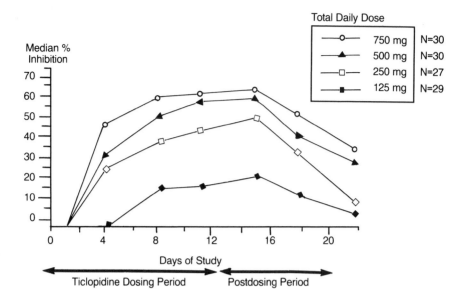

FIGURE 4.6. Percent inhibition of ADP-induced platelet aggregation by days in study: high ADP concentration (ICM 1687).

in vitro to PRP from ticlopidine-dosed volunteers, had no effect on inhibition of platelet aggregation by ticlopidine (Table 4.5). The small increase seen in cAMP after ticlopidine treatment compared with pretreatment may result from inhibition of platelet activation that often occurs during phlebotomy.

Platelet Activation by ADP

At current clinical doses, ticlopidine inhibition is exhibited primarily after ADP-mediated activation of platelet aggregation. Ticlopidine inhibits aggrega-

TABLE 4.5. Effect of SQ-22536 on platelet aggregation[1] inhibited by ticlopidine treatment.

Group	N	Transmittance change (%) (mean ± SD)	Percent inhibition of aggregation (mean ± SD)
Predose	13	67.5 ± 7.9	
Ticlopidine[2]	13	25.5 ± 15.8	65 ± 21
Ticlopidine + SQ-225362	13	25.0 ± 14.7	66 ± 20

[1] Aggregation induced by ADP (5–10 μM).
[2] PRP obtained 12 hours after last dose (250 mg, bid, for 4 days). Inhibition calculated against each individual's predose values. SQ-22536 added in vitro to PRP to give a concentration of 0.3 μM.

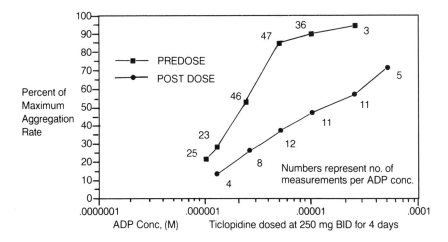

FIGURE 4.7. The inhibition of initial rate of human platelet aggregation: ADP dose-response effect (ICM 830).

tion of platelets, stimulated directly by ADP (Figure 4.7) or indirectly by ADP, released from platelet granules by other inducers.[34,35] As discussed above, ADP is an important physiologic inducer of platelet aggregation mediated via platelet membrane GPIIb/IIIa (Figure 4.3, Step 7). Irreversible platelet aggregation requires fibrinogen binding to this exposed receptor. Absence of the receptor for fibrinogen binding results in severe bleeding disorders.[15-17] Similarly, inhibiting exposure of this receptor results in markedly prolonged bleeding time measurements (Table 4.2).

Aspirin at concentrations that completely block platelet thromboxane synthesis in vitro does not inhibit ADP-induced binding of fibrinogen to platelets and thus has no effect on expression of the fibrinogen receptor on platelet membrane GPIIb/IIIa.[36,37] On the other hand, after oral treatment with ticlopidine (250 mg, bid) for 7 days, ADP-induced fibrinogen binding to human platelets is inhibited more than 85% (Figure 4.8). Seven days after cessation of ticlopidine treatment, ADP-induced platelet–fibrinogen binding is still significantly inhibited (p < 0.01). This long duration of inhibition of ADP-induced platelet fibrinogen binding is another indication of ticlopidine's irreversible effect on platelet function. Ticlopidine's ability to inhibit fibrinogen binding to platelets supports its use for aspirin-resistant thromboembolic disease.

Studies have been done to determine whether inhibition of fibrinogen binding by ticlopidine is associated with quantitative or qualitative alteration of the GPIIb/IIIa. No changes in this platelet heterodimer are found after ticlopidine treatment using crossed immunoelectrophoresis or reactivity of several antibodies to GPIIb/IIIa compared with pretreatment behavior.[38,39] It is concluded

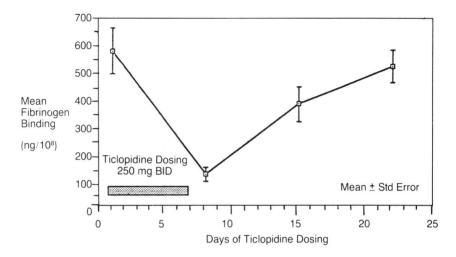

FIGURE 4.8. The inhibition of fibrinogen binding to human platelets stimulated by ADP after ticlopidine treatment of healthy volunteers.

that there is no direct evidence that ticlopidine alters the platelet membrane glycoprotein on which the fibrinogen receptor is located.

It has been observed that neither the ADP-induced platelet shape change,[40] nor the incorporation of 5'-fluorosulfonylbenzoyl adenosine,[41] an affinity label for aggregin (a putative platelet receptor for ADP), are inhibited after treatment with ticlopidine or its analogs, PCR 4099 and clopidogrel. These observations suggest that ticlopidine does not inhibit binding of ADP to its receptor.

Reports from several investigators who have studied the effect of treatment with ticlopidine on Ca^{2+} fluxes in platelets after stimulation with inducers are mixed. Whereas Derian and Friedman[42] found that both ADP- and thrombin-induced calcium mobilization were inhibited, neither of two other laboratories[38,40] were able to confirm this finding. It seems likely that demonstrating inhibition of calcium mobilization requires higher doses of ticlopidine than used in those studies.

The general conclusion that can be drawn from the above reports is that ticlopidine acts by inhibiting signal transduction and not by altering either platelet ADP receptors or GPIIb/IIIa.

Summary of Ticlopidine's Mechanism of Action

The molecular mechanism whereby ticlopidine inhibits platelet activation remains unknown. However, certain characteristics of this mechanism have been established. Ticlopidine's primary action is to inhibit the binding of fibrinogen to platelets, and ticlopidine's inhibition of platelet function is irreversible for the life of the platelet. Platelet aggregation inhibition of ticlopidine does not depend upon a circulating metabolite but does require some as yet unknown metabolism-dependent alterations of platelets in vivo. Ticlopidine does not inhibit cyclooxy-genase or cAMP phosphodiesterase, and platelet aggregation inhibition by ticlopidine does not depend on elevation of platelet cAMP. At this time, the most likely explanation for the action of ticlopidine is that it inhibits signal transduction initiated by agonists causing platelet aggregation.

References

1. Harker LA. Pathogenesis of thrombosis. In Williams WJ (ed), *Hematology*, 4th ed. McGraw-Hill, New York, 1990, pp 1559–1569.
2. Harker LA. Antithrombotic therapy. In Williams WJ (ed), *Hematology*, 4th ed. McGraw-Hill, New York, 1990, pp 1569–1581.
3. Haerem JW. Platelet aggregates in intramyocardial vessels of patients dying suddenly and unexpectedly of coronary artery disease. *Atherosclerosis* 1972;**15**:199–213.
4. Antiplatelet Trialists Collaboration. Secondary prevention of vascular disease by prolonged antiplatelet treatment. *Br Med J* 1988;**296**:320.
5. The Aspirin Myocardial Infarction Study Research Group. A randomized, controlled trial of aspirin in persons recovered from myocardial infarction. *JAMA* 1980;**243**:661–669.
6. The Persantine-Aspirin Reinfarction Study Research Group. Persantine and aspirin in coronary heart disease. *Circulation* 1980;**62**:449–461.
7. The Anturane Reinfarction Trial Research Group. Sulfinpyrazone in the prevention of cardiac death after myocardial infarction. The Anturane Reinfarction Trial. *N Eng J Med* 1978;**282**:289–295.
8. Canadian Cooperative Study Group. A randomized trial of aspirin and sulfinpyrazone in threatened stroke. *N Eng J Med* 1978;**299**:53–59.
9. Lewis HD, Davis JW, Archibald DG, Steinke WE, Smitheran TC, Doherty JE, et al. Protective effects of aspirin against acute myocardial infarction and death in men with unstable angina. *N Eng J Med* 1983;**309(7)**:398–403.
10. Antiplatelet Trialist Collaboration. Secondary prevention of vascular disease by prolonged antiplatelet treatment. *Br Med J* 1988;**296**:320–331.
11. Gaarder A, Jonsen J, Laland S, Hellem A, Owren PA. Adenosine diphosphate in red cells as a factor in the adhesiveness of human blood platelets. *Nature* 1964;**202**:909–910.
12. Born GVR, Bergquist D, Arfors K-E. Evidence for inhibition of platelet activation in blood by a drug effect on erythrocytes. *Nature* 1976;**259**:233–235.
13. Zawilska KM, Born GVR, Begent NA. Effect of ADP-utilizing enzymes on the arterial bleeding time in rats and rabbits. *Br J Haematol* 1982;**50**:317–325.
14. Begent NA, Born GVR. Growth rate in vivo of platelet thrombi, produced by iontophoresis of ADP, as a function on mean blood flow velocity. *Nature* (London) 1970;**227**:926–930.
15. Bennett JS, Vilaire G. Exposure of platelet fibrinogen receptors by ADP and epinephrine. *J Clin Invest* 1979;**64**:1393–1401.
16. Zucker MB, Pert JH, Hilgartner MW. Platelet function in a patient with thrombasthenia. *Blood* 1966;**28**:524–534.

17. Caen JP, Castaldi PA, Leclerc JC, et al. Congenital bleeding disorders with long bleeding time and normal platelet count. I. Glanzmann's thrombasthenia (report of 15 patients). *Am J Med* 1966;**41**:4–26.
18. Malmsten C, Hamberg M, Svensson J, Samuelsson B. Physiological role of an endoperoxide in human platelets: hemostatic defect due to platelet cyclooxygenase deficiency. *Proc Nat Acad Sci* USA 1975;**72(4)**:1446–1450.
19. Teitelbaum P, Smith S. Detailed summary: the absorption, distribution, metabolism, excretion, and pharmacokinetics of ticlopidine hydrochloride in animals. *NDA* 19-979 1989;**759**:9–13.
20. Teitelbaum P, Shah J. Detailed summary: absorption, distribution, metabolism, excretion, and pharmacokinetics of ticlopidine hydrochloride in humans. *NDA* 19-979 1989;**761**:8–10.
21. Gent M, Blakely JA, Easton JD, Ellis DJ, Hachinski VC, Harbison JW, Panak EA, Roberts RS, Sicurella J, Turpie AG. The Canadian American Ticlopidine Study (CATS) in thromboembolic stroke. *Lancet* 1989;**1**:1215–1220.
22. Ashida S, Abiko Y. Inhibition of platelet aggregation by a new agent, ticlopidine. *Thromb Haemost* 1978;**40**:542–550.
23. di Minno G, Cerbone AM, Mattioli PL, Turco S, Iovine C, Mancini M. Functionally thrombasthenic state in normal platelets following administration of ticlopidine. *J Clin Invest* 1985;**75**:328–338.
24. Bruno JJ, Chang L, McSpadden MM, Yang D. The effect of oral ticlopidine on arachidonic acid products in human platelets. *Agents Actions Suppl* 1984;**15**:76–87.
25. Rao AK, Willis J, Holmsen H. A major role of ADP in thromboxane transfer experiments: studies in patients with platelet secretion defects. *J Lab Clin Med* 1984;**104**:116–126.
26. Hanson SR, Harker LA. Baboon models of acute arterial thrombosis. *Thromb Haemost* 1987;**58**:801–805.
27. Ashida S, Abiko Y. Mode of action of ticlopidine in inhibition of platelet aggregation in the rat. *Thromb Haemost* 1979;**41(2)**:436–449.
28. Ashida S, Abiko Y. Mode of action of ticlopidine in inhibition of platelet aggregation in the rat. *Thromb Haemost* 1979;**41(2)**:436–449.
29. Bruno JJ, Taylor LA, Feamster C. Role of platelet cAMP and prostaglandin synthesis in platelet inhibition by ticlopidine hydrochloride. *Thromb Haemost* 1981;**46(1)**:66.
30. Bonne C, Battais E. Ticlopidine and adenylate cyclase. *Agents Actions Suppl* 1984;**15**:88–96.
31. Alvarez R, Lundell GR, Bruno JJ. Cyclic AMP accumulation in human platelets in response to prostaglandin E1: effect of oral administration of ticlopidine. Quo Vadis? Ticlopidine, Montpelier 20–21, October 1983:76–79.
32. Defreyn G, Gachet C, Savi P, Driot F, Cazenave JP, Maffrand JP. Ticlopidine and clopidogrel (SR 25990C) selectively neutralize ADP inhibition of PGE1-activated platelet adenylate cyclase in rats and rabbits. *Thromb Haemost* 1991;**65(2)**:186–190.
33. Puri RN, Mills DCB, Hu C-J, Minniti C, Grana G, Freedman M, Freedman S, Colman RF, Colman RW. Clopidogrel, a ticlopidine analog, impairs the interaction of ADP with the receptor mediating adenyl cyclase without altering the modification of aggregin. *Clin Res* 1991;**39(2)**:366A.
34. Bernat A, Vallée E, Maffrand JP, Gordon JL. The role of platelets and ADP in experimental thrombosis induced by venous stasis in the rat. *Thromb Res* 1988;**52**:65–70.

35. Maffrand JP, Defreyn G, Bernat A, Delebassée D, Tissinier AM. Reviewed pharmacology of ticlopidine. *Angiologie Suppl* 1988;**77(5)**:6–13.
36. Chang L, Bruno JJ. Effect of orally administered ticlopidine on ADP-induced binding of fibrinogen to platelets. Quo Vadis? Ticlopidine, Montpelier 20–21, October 1983: 90–94.
37. Bennett JS, Vilaire G, Burch JW. A role for prostaglandins and thromboxanes in the exposure of platelet fibrinogen receptors. *J Clin Invest* 1981;**68**:981–987.
38 Hardisty RM, Powling MJ, Nokes TJC. The action of ticlopidine on human platelets: studies on aggregation, secretion, calcium mobilization and membrane glycoproteins. *Thromb Haemost* 1990;**64(1)**:105–155.
39. Gachet C, Stierle A, Cazenave JP, Ohlmann P, Lanza F, Bouloux C, Maffrand JP. The thienopyridine PCR 4099 selectively inhibits ADP-induced platelet aggregation and fibrinogen binding without modifying the membrane glycoprotein IIbIIIa complex in rat and in man. *Biochem Pharmacol* 1990;**40(2)**:229–238.
40. Féliste R, Simon MF, Chap H, Douste-Blazy L, Defreyn G, Maffrand JP. Effect of PCR 4099 on ADP-induced calcium movements and phospatidic acid production in rat platelets. *Biochem Pharmacol* 1988;**37(13)**:2559–2564.
41. Puri RN, Mills DCB, Hu C-J, Minniti C, Grana G, Freedman M, Freedman S, Colman RF, Colman RW. Clopidogrel, a ticlopidine analog, impairs the interactions of ADP with the receptor mediating adenyl cyclase without altering the modification of aggregin. *Clin Res* 1991;**39(2)**:366A.
42. Derian CK, Friedman PA. Effect of ticlopidine ex vivo on platelet intracellular calcium mobilization. *Thromb Res* 1988;**50**:65–76.

5
Clinical Studies of Stroke Prevention with Ticlopidine in Man

WILLIAM PRYSE-PHILLIPS

Introduction

Lawrence Craven's plaintive reports from his Glendale general practice in the 1950s[1,2] were generally ignored until Barnett and his Canadian collaborators demonstrated in the late 1970s that aspirin indeed reduces the risk of completed stroke following transient ischemic attack (TIA) or minor stroke. Since then, the concept that stroke is the inevitable sentence of an angry Providence has withered in the light of scientific inquiry into the causes of, and the potential remedies for, this often devastating affliction. Various drugs having effects on platelets have been examined. Some have been shown potent in preventing subsequent strokes, some impotent. An overview analysis of their effects in preventing major vascular events due to atherothrombosis is presented in Chapter 8. This chapter will review the clinical studies of stroke prevention with ticlopidine. Before they are considered, a note on the context of the disease is appropriate.

Natural History of Stroke

After a TIA, an increased risk of stroke is incurred, running at about 5%/year, with the hazard being greatest in the first year and *a fortiori* in the first week after the TIA.[3] The early mortality rate is about 6%/year which is worse than the 3–4% annual rate in patients with angina pectoris. After atherothrombotic brain infarcts (ABIs), nearly 10% of subjects will suffer another stroke each year thereafter; but in both of these groups the greater risk of dying is from cardiac causes rather than stroke. Figures such as these compel one to consider what can be done to reduce the mortality consequent upon such morbidity.

Antiplatelet Agents

Scientific inquiry is designed to provide simple and useful answers. However, not uniquely, our present state of knowledge regarding antiplatelet agents and strokes is substantially incomplete. We may begin with an undisputed truth: fewer vascular events occur in a population in which the subjects' platelets are paralyzed. How can this be parlayed into a reasonable scheme for stroke prevention?

The Ticlopidine-Aspirin Stroke Study (TASS)[4]

TASS was designed to test the beneficial and adverse effects of ticlopidine compared to aspirin in the prevention of stroke and death in patients with TIA and minor stroke.

In order to recruit the 3000 patients needed to detect a significant beneficial effect of ticlopidine over aspirin, 56 centers in the United States and Canada contributed patients over a period of 5.8 years from February 1982. Patient entry criteria included occurrence of TIA, transient monocular blindness (TMB), reversible ischemic neurological deficit (RIND), or minor stroke with 80% recovery during the previous 3 months. Patients excluded from the study were: those less than 40 years old; women of childbearing potential; those having symptoms considered to be secondary to vasospasm, cardiogenic embolism, or hematological disorders; those with previous aspirin intolerance; those who needed continued use of aspirin or anticoagulants; or those suffering from other diseases or mental abnormality threatening their ability to continue participation for the duration of the trial.

Baseline studies were performed to screen for such disorders, and CT scanning of the head and arteriography were performed if indicated clinically. The entry criteria of each patient, and every event occurring during the trial, were scrutinized by an independent neurologist who was unaware of the treatment allocations. Ingestion of all known platelet-inhibiting drugs was prohibited. All patients were followed to the conclusion of the trial, whether or not they were still taking the study drug. Reasons for premature termination were recorded, and a primary reason assigned by the masked reviewer.

Patients were randomly assigned to treatment with either ticlopidine (250 mg twice daily) or aspirin (650 mg twice daily) packaged identically. Randomization in each center was stratified on the basis of a history of ischemic cardiovascular disease, occurrence of a moderate stroke over the 3 months before entry, and gender. All patients were clinically evaluated by a neurologist 1 month after entry and every 4 months thereafter. Compliance was assessed by tablet counts. Patients, investigators, adjudicators, and sponsor remained unaware of treatment allocations. These were known only to an independent external safety committee and the independent randomizing research institute. Adjudication as to entry and endpoint events used prepared criteria to ensure accuracy and consistency. The primary endpoint was death or nonfatal stroke (thus including fatal strokes as well); secondary endpoints included the first fatal and nonfatal stroke.

TABLE 5.1. Relative risk reduction for major endpoints.

	% reduction ticlopidine vs. aspirin		
	1 year	2 years	3 years
Stroke and death	42	18	13
Stroke and stroke death	47	22	21
All cardio- and cerebrovascular mortality, myocardial infarct and stroke	39	15	10

Results

Of 8814 patients screened, 5745 did not satisfy entry criteria for the following reasons: symptoms were due to other disorders: patients were thought unlikely to survive 5 years; a severe completed stroke had occurred within the last 3 months; aspirin hypersensitivity (280 patients); or peptic ulceration (226 patients). A further 22% of potentially eligible patients declined to participate, and 13% were excluded because they underwent elective carotid endarterectomy. Of the 3069 eligible patients randomized, 1529 were assigned to ticlopidine, of which 1518 took the drug. Of the 1540 assigned to aspirin, 1527 took it. Men comprised two-thirds of the study population. The average age was 63.9 years (range 39–94 years). Patients' baseline characteristics did not differ between the two groups.

Of the qualifying ischemic events, 70% were judged to be in the carotid territory, 25% vertebrobasilar, and in the remainder the localization was uncertain. Cerebral arteriography was performed in 51% of the patients and was abnormal in 60% of these. CT scans were performed in 75% of cases; half showed abnormalities.

Good compliance was attained as nearly 90% of the patients took at least 75% of the medication for 90% of the time. Forty-six patients taking ticlopidine and 38 taking aspirin were lost to follow-up by the end of the trial. Fifty-two percent of the patients taking ticlopidine and 47% of those taking aspirin stopped treatment before that time. The mean duration of ticlopidine therapy was 778 ± 603 days and for aspirin was 858 ± 582 days.

Using intention-to-treat analysis, ticlopidine achieved a 21% relative stroke risk reduction (95% CI-4 to 38%; $p < 0.05$) and a 12% risk reduction in non-fatal stroke or vascular death when compared to aspirin (95% CI-2 to 26%; $p = 0.02$). Using efficacy analysis (but spanning the whole of the follow-up period), 164 patients on ticlopidine and 220 on aspirin experienced one of the primary outcome events (death from any cause or nonfatal stroke). Cumulative event rates at 12, 24, and 36 months (Table 5.1) showed risk reductions in favor of ticlopidine, women having a better outcome than men, although this reduction diminished over the 3-year period.

Fatal or nonfatal strokes occurred in 111 patients on ticlopidine and in 165 on aspirin, the cumulative event rate showing a significant benefit in favor of

TABLE 5.2. Therapeutic effectiveness of ticlopidine (TASS).

Endpoint	Intent-to-treat analysis[1]			Efficacy analysis[2]		
	% reduction in risk[3]	Cumulative event rates per 100 (TIC, ASA)	P-value[4]	% reduction in risk[3]	Cumulative event rates per 100 (TIC, ASA)	P-value[4]
Death from all causes or nonfatal stroke						
1 year	41.1	5.2 8.8	0.048	42.0	4.6 7.9	0.048
2 years	20.2	11.6 14.6		18.3	10.3 12.6	
3 years	12.0	17.0 19.4		NA	14.5 15.6	
Fatal or nonfatal stroke						
1 year	46.2	3.4 6.2	0.024	47.6	3.4 6.4	0.011
2 years	25.7	7.4 9.9		22.2	7.6 9.8	
3 years	21.3	10.0 12.7		20.5	10.3 13.0	
Overall reduction[5]	21			27		

[1] Includes all randomized patients and all events.
[2] Includes truly eligible patients and only events occurring on medication.
[3] Reduction by ticlopidine (TIC) over aspirin (ASA).
[4] Based on Mantel-Haenszel test of the Kaplan-Meier time-to-event curves.
[5] Estimate of constant reduction in risk based on Cox proportional hazards model.

ticlopidine (p = 0.01), again more obviously in women. Relative reductions in the main endpoints were seen throughout the trial, but the figures diminished (Table 5.2). Distribution, type, and severity of the first stroke suffered were similar in the two groups, most being atherothrombotic and in the carotid arterial territory.

Neither an increase nor decrease in the number of fatal or nonfatal myocardial infarctions occurred in the ticlopidine group during the trial.

Subgroup analyses of the cumulative event rates for the primary and secondary endpoints, based upon age, sex, prior history of stroke, hypertension or diabetes, cardiac failure or peripheral vascular disease, inconclusively suggested that ticlopidine was superior in benefits to aspirin in all of these categories.

Comment

For the apparent reduction in efficacy of the drugs over the 3 years, two reasons may be adduced. First, the risk of stroke is far greater in the first year than in either of the next two. There was, as a result, less room for superior results to be displayed. Second, those that were destined to suffer a stroke were likely to do so earlier, so the population in whom risk reduction was being sought was one which was progressively less likely to have a stroke and was also decreasing in size. Since the greatest need for prevention of ischemic stroke is in the early period after TIA or other warning, this emphatic early response to ticlopidine is an important point in favor of using the drug, accentuating the overall relative superiority of ticlopidine over aspirin shown in this study.

The Canadian-American Ticlopidine Study (CATS)[5]

CATS was designed to test the beneficial and adverse effects of ticlopidine compared to *placebo* in the prevention of stroke, myocardial infarction, and vascular death in patients with a recent major stroke.

Although the pathogeneses of TIA and severe atherothrombotic brain infarction overlap, the effect of antiplatelet drugs has been examined more often, and shown to be of value mostly in TIAs and minor strokes. Less than 20% of thromboembolic stroke are preceded by TIAs while the rate of subsequent stroke, myocardial infarction, or vascular death following recovery from thromboembolic stroke has been reported as nearly 20% at the 1st year and about 25% after 2 years.[6] A study of ticlopidine's effect in the prevention of recurrent stroke was therefore appropriate, and in the absence of evidence of benefit from single studies of other treatments, it was possible to employ a placebo control. While CATS was in progress, a Swedish trial of high-dose aspirin vs. placebo following completed stroke did not show any benefit for aspirin.[7]

Where TASS studied the milder end of the spectrum of cerebrovascular disease, the CATS trial was concerned with the more seriously ill patient. In this trial, 1053 patients recruited from 25 study centers in North America having thromboembolic stroke more than 1 week but less than 4 months before entry (including atherothrombotic and lacunar infarctions but not cardioembolic infarcts) were evaluated for a mean period of 2 years. Patients excluded were those: likely to remain bedridden or who were demented; with severe comorbid conditions, drug abuse or alcoholism; unable to take ticlopidine; in whom the qualifying stroke was secondary to angiography or endarterectomy; or considered to require long-term anticoagulant or antiplatelet therapy. Patients entered but later determined to be truly ineligible were reported but were not included.

Eligible patients were randomly allocated to receive ticlopidine 250 mg twice daily or identical placebo and were followed up at 1 and 4 months after entry and every 4 months thereafter to a maximum of 3 years. Local and central laboratory monitoring, as well as testing of compliance by pill counts from study medication bottles, were performed at each visit. Thus compliance and other coordination aspects of the study, including blinding, verification, and adjudication methods, closely resembled those employed in TASS.

The primary outcome events for the efficacy assessment were the most common and most serious clinical events in patients with atherosclerotic disease, namely nonfatal stroke, nonfatal myocardial infarction, and vascular death. Secondary endpoints were fatal and nonfatal stroke and, to allow comparisons with TASS, deaths from all causes plus nonfatal stroke. Subarachnoid hemorrhage and primary intracerebral hemorrhage were not included as primary outcomes. These, however, were analyzed separately.

Results

Of 1072 patients entered who were randomly allocated to ticlopidine or placebo, 19 were ruled truly ineligible by adjudicators blind to the treatment. Average follow-up was 24 months, and the mean time patients were on the study drug was 19 months (placebo) and 17 months (ticlopidine). Four patients (three on ticlopidine and one on placebo) were irretrievably lost to follow-up. The rate of early permanent discontinuation of the study drug was 40% in the placebo group and 52% in the ticlopidine group. A summary compilation of the therapeutic effectiveness of cumulative event rates in the 2 groups, and the relative reduction in events of ticlopidine over placebo is shown in Table 5.3.

Recurrence of stroke was the most frequent first outcome event. For the primary group of first vascular outcomes (1053 patients), there were 188 events in the placebo group during 773 patient-years at risk, and average rate of 15.3%/year. There were 74 events in the ticlopidine group during 683 patient-years at risk, an average rate of 10.8%/year. Ticlopidine thus provided a relative risk reduction on treatment of 30.2% (95% CI 7.5 to 48.3; p = 0.006) in the incidence of stroke, myocardial infarction, or vascular death: 28.1% for men (p = 0.037) and 32.4% for women (p = 0.045). A subgroup analysis comparing the relative efficacy of ticlopidine for the two types of qualifying stroke (i.e.,

TABLE 5.3. Therapeutic effectiveness of ticlopidine (CATS).

Endpoint	Intent-to-treat analysis[1]			Efficacy analysis[2]		
	% reduction in risk[3]	Cumulative event rates per 100 (TIC, PLA)	P-value[4]	% reduction in risk[3]	Cumulative event rates per 100 (TIC, PLA)	P-value[4]
Vascular death, nonfatal stroke or nonfatal MI						
1 year	31.6	11.2 16.4	0.049	36.9	10.4 16.5	0.014
2 years	18.9	20.0 24.7		23.1	19.3 25.1	
3 years	14.2	27.7 32.2		24.5	24.4 32.3	
Overall reduction[5]	23.3			30.2		
Death from all causes or nonfatal stroke						
1 year	26.8	12.5 17.0	0.173	38.4	10.3 16.7	0.032
2 years	11.4	24.4 27.5		19.3	20.9 25.9	
3 years	4.7	32.9 34.6		8.6	28.8 31.5	
Overall reduction[5]	22			27		
Fatal or nonfatal stroke						
1 year	30.2	8.8 12.6		33.4	8.3 12.4	0.017
2 years	26.1	14.5 19.6		33.6	13.2 19.9	
3 years	5.2	22.0 23.2		24.3	18.6 24.6	
Overall reduction[5]	22			33.5		

[1] Includes all randomized patients and all events.
[2] Includes truly eligible patients and only events occurring on medication.
[3] Reduction by ticlopidine (TIC) over placebo (PLA).
[4] Based on Mantel-Haenszel test of the Kaplan-Meier time-to-event curves.
[5] Estimate of constant reduction in risk based on Cox proportional hazards model.

atherothrombotic and lacunar) showed the risk reductions to be similar. For the secondary endpoint of fatal and nonfatal stroke, the on treatment risk reduction of ticlopidine was 33.5%.

Ticlopidine's benefits were consistent and greatest when the outcomes were restricted to vascular events. However, the benefit persisted with the addition of nonvascular deaths, the relative risk reduction then being 24.1% (p = 0.023). Recurrence of stroke was more common in the placebo than in the ticlopidine group (p = 0.008), and the distribution of severity among these strokes was similar, as was the type of stroke. Of the 143 recurrences of stroke, 111 (78%) were atherothrombotic, 28 (20%) were lacunar infarctions, and 4 (2%) were cardioembolic; 83% of patients with these outcome events had a CT or MR brain scan.

An intention-to-treat analysis, based on all eligible patients and all outcome events showed a 23.3% relative risk reduction in the cluster of stroke, myocardial infarction, or vascular death (95% CI 1.0 to 40.5; p = 0.02), confirming the benefit of ticlopidine.

An adverse experience was reported at some time during the course of the study in 283 (54%) patients in the ticlopidine group and in 181 (34%) taking placebo. Such experiences were reported as severe in 43 (8.2%) and 15 (2.8%) patients in the ticlopidine and placebo groups, respectively (p = 0.001), for an excess of 5.4% on ticlopidine. Sixty-two (11.8%) and 15 (2.8%) taking ticlopidine and placebo, respectively, discontinued the drug permanently due to unwanted effects. Neutropenia was the most serious of these. Two patients in the placebo group had subarachnoid hemorrhages (both fatal), and two patients in the ticlopidine group had primary intracerebral hemorrhages, one of which was fatal.

Comment

The CATS trial shows that ticlopidine reduces the incidence of subsequent stroke, myocardial infarction, and vascular death in patients surviving a moderate or severe thromboembolic stroke. The overall relative reduction in risk of the major vascular outcomes was 23.3% (CI 1.0 to 40.5; p = 0.20) in the intent-to-treat analysis and 30.2% (CI 7.5 to 48.3; p = 0.006) in the efficacy analysis. The efficacy analysis was based only on patients with the disease of interest, including the major vascular outcomes of stroke, myocardial infarction, and vascular death, but excluding nonvascular deaths and any events occurring more than 28 days after the study drug was permanently discontinued. This analysis increases clinical relevance by excluding events and patients that were unlikely to be affected by the treatment. The rules and procedures for making decisions about such exclusions were published in a paper submitted before the treatment code was broken.[8] Furthermore, no bias resulted from excluding ineligible patients or events after patients discontinued their study drugs. Confidence in ticlopidine's efficacy is further strengthened by its consistency of

TABLE 5.4. Unwanted effects (TASS, efficacy group).

	Ticlopidine	Aspirin
Patients exposed	1518	1527
	Number (%)	
Diarrhea	310 (20.4)	150 (9.8)
Dyspepsia	191 (12.6)	210 (13.8)
Gastrointestinal bleeding	7 (0.5)	21 (1.4)
Gastritis	13 (0.9)	26 (1.7)
Peptic ulcer	12 (0.8)	45 (2.9)
Rash	180 (12.9)	80 (5.2)
Severe neutropenia	13 (0.9)	0

Note: These figures resemble, and are in general representative of, the figures reported in ATS.

benefit in different centers for the two types of qualifying stroke (atherothrom-botic or lacunar infarcts), for men and women, and when based on an intention-to-treat or efficacy analysis.

Unwanted Effects in TASS and CATS

This subject is reviewed in detail in Chapter 9 and will be discussed only briefly here. Overall in TASS, 62% of patients experienced some untoward reaction during the trial. Diarrhea was noted in 20% of patients on ticlopidine and 10% of those on aspirin. Trial medication was permanently discontinued for this reason in 6.4% of the former and in 1.8% of the latter group, although a temporary reduction in dosage was often sufficient to relieve it. Although 506 (9%) of the 5475 patients screened for TASS could not be randomized because of aspirin intolerance or gastrointestinal bleeding in the previous 2 years; peptic ulceration, gastritis or gastrointestinal bleeding occurred in 2.2% of patients on ticlopidine and 6.2% of patients on aspirin. Two deaths occurred in the aspirin group after hematemesis. Other gastrointestinal adverse effects were common in both groups (Tables 5.4 and 5.5).

TABLE 5.5. Gastrointestinal adverse effects in TASS and CATS.

	Ticlopidine	ASA	Placebo
No. patients exposed to study medication	2048	1527	536
Adverse Experience	(Percentages)		
Peptic ulcer	0.6	2.8	—
Hemorrhagic complication	1.5	3.1	—

Other bleeding events, such as purpura, petechiae, easy bruising, epistaxis, and microscopic hematuria, occurred in 9% of patients on ticlopidine and 10% of those on aspirin.

Maculopapular or urticarial rashes developed in 11.9% of patients on ticlopidine and 5.2% of those on aspirin. Although none was life-threatening, ticlopidine was discontinued for this reason in 3.4% and aspirin in 0.8% of patients, always with prompt resolution of the rash.

Severe neutropenia (absolute neutrophil count 450/mm^3) developed in eight white women and five white men taking ticlopidine between 1 and 3 months after starting the drug, but cell counts returned to normal within 2 weeks of stopping ingestion. Mild to moderate neutropenia (absolute neutrophil count 450–1200/mm^3) occurred in 22 patients on ticlopidine and in 12 on aspirin.

Patients on ticlopidine in TASS showed an increase in total plasma cholesterol levels from month 1, stabilizing to a mean increase of 11% over the initial (usually elevated) level by month 4, while the increase in aspirin-treated patients was 2%. The ratio of HDL to total cholesterol did not change. The profile of unwanted effects was identical in CATS and in other smaller studies reported.

Other Studies of Ticlopidine in Cerebrovascular Disease

Eight smaller trials of ticlopidine vs. aspirin in the primary or secondary prevention of stroke have been conducted in patients with cerebrovascular disease, seven of them in Japan. Only three in all were double-blind and randomized, all lasted a year or less, and the total number of patients entered was less than 800.

The overall conclusions from a review of these small trials is that their value is limited, but in the aggregate ticlopidine was superior to aspirin, much as was shown in the TASS trial. One small, double-blind trial in Japan[9] compared the effects of ticlopidine (200 mg daily) and aspirin (500 mg daily), each with placebo tablets added over a 12-month period in 334 patients who had TIAs in the previous three months. Efficacy analysis in 281 of these subjects showed no reduction in TIA, but there was a non-significant reduction in small strokes, myocardial infarctions, and completed strokes combined, although only 5 patients developed cerebral infarcts. The study continued unblinded in 131 of these patients for a further 24 months. Review of the results over the whole period showed that at 3 years, subjects taking ticlopidine had fewer (34 vs. 52) cerebrovascular events than those taking aspirin, although only the difference in the cumulative incidence of events over the whole 3-year period attained statistical significance (p = 0.036). Incidence of myocardial infarction and of intracerebral hemorrhage were similar in the two groups.

The Ticlopidine Microangiopathy of Diabetes study (TIMAD)[10] was a randomized, doubly-masked, placebo-controlled trial designed to assess the effect of ticlopidine in reducing progression of non-proliferative diabetic retinopathy in 435 patients with insulin-dependent diabetes mellitus over 3 years.

The mean yearly increase in definite microaneurysms shown by fluorescein angiograms was lower (p = 0.03) in the ticlopidine group. The drug yielded a seven-fold reduction in the yearly microaneurysm progression score compared with placebo (p = 0.03). Development of new vessels in the ticlopidine group was not significantly reduced, but the overall progression of retinopathy was less marked (p = 0.04). It was noted that the greatest inhibition of platelet aggregation was associated with cessation or reversal of microaneurysm progression, indicating an effect of the drug not only at the arterial, but also at the arteriolar level.

Studies of Ticlopidine in Combination

Uchiyama[11] conducted the first trial of ticlopidine for secondary prevention of TIA, using a dose of 200 mg per day (the usual dose in Japan), enough to suppress platelet aggregation in the average Japanese. The report demonstrated that the incidence of ischemic events was reduced by ticlopidine and that platelet aggregation induced by ADP was inhibited in patients with multiple episodes of TIA or RIND. In a subsequent double-blind, multicenter trial of ticlopidine vs. aspirin in patients with TIAs,[12] reduction in the incidence of subsequent stroke and myocardial infarction was significantly greater in patients treated with 200 mg of ticlopidine that in those treated with 500 mg of aspirin at 12 and 36 months after entry.

The relation between stroke recurrence and platelet aggregation in patients treated with aspirin or ticlopidine was investigated by Sato.[13] Platelet aggregation induced by ADP was significantly inhibited after administration of these drugs in the group of patients without recurrence, but not in the group of patients who had a recurrent stroke. However, stroke still recurred despite the inhibition of platelet aggregation induced by ADP in some patients, which was thought to be due to the presence of intact pathways for platelet aggregation via ADP, arachidonic acid, or PAF, although this could not be proven since platelet aggregation induced by arachidonic acid and PAF was not measured in that study.

Uchiyama[14] used combination therapy with aspirin plus ticlopidine in a further trial involving 72 patients. He reported that the combination inhibited platelet aggregation by PAF, ADP, and arachidonic acid and markedly reduced the plasma concentration of TG and PF4, whereas either drug alone did not affect or only slightly reduced them. He concluded that aspirin plus ticlopidine can suppress *in vivo* platelet secretion that cannot be suppressed when only one or two of the pathways leading to platelet aggregation is inhibited by either drug alone. The combination produced a greater prolongation of bleeding time (and more hemorrhagic complications) than did either agent alone. This is additional evidence that the combination can inhibit *in vivo* platelet function by inhibiting most pathways leading to platelet aggregation. Moreover, platelet survival was prolonged and platelet lysis was reduced after treatment with both drugs despite the fact that neither measure of platelet function was significantly altered after treatment with either alone. The combination of low dose aspirin and ticlopidine was thus considered to be a potent antiplatelet strategy, although the clinical importance of the changes observed were not described. Indeed, the combination may prove to be toxic.

Discussion

The results of drug trials are usually reported in one or both of two ways. Intention-to-treat analyses use all the patients randomized, even if they are later deemed ineligible, are withdrawn for any reason, do not take the medication or are improperly assessed. They incorporate these known biases in an effort to correct for any potential biases in favor of the drug introduced by later withdrawal of patients and inform about the likely effect of the drug across a whole practice. Such biases would be intolerable if introduced in an effort to make a test drug apparently more effective. Efficacy (or on-treatment) analyses report the results in those patients who actually have the disease of interest and take the drug appropriately, and in whom full results are available. In the TASS and CATS studies, events occurring during a period (10 days in TASS and 28 days in CATS) after stopping the medication were also included. In the CATS, the reduction in incidence of stroke among patients taking ticlopidine was not significant by intention-to-treat analysis (p = 0.06) but was (p = 0.017) by efficacy analysis. The difference lies in the patients included in the intention-to-treat analysis who were included even though they had not taken ticlopidine for over 28 days when an event occurred or had been improperly included in the trial in the first place because they did not fulfill inclusion criteria.

Which method of analysis to accept is arguable. For example, if in a trial of penicillin for streptococcal infection, a quarter of the patients were allergic to it and another quarter actually had *E. coli* infections, then it is likely that intention-to-treat analysis would show that penicillin was ineffective for strepto-coccal infections, which is clearly not the case. Since efficacy analyses inform about clinical pharmacology—the expected effect of the drug in subjects who take it and have the disease that can respond to it—it seems appropriate when investigating the effect of a new agent to use this method as well as the intention-to-treat analysis.

The aspirin dose employed in the TASS trial was mandated by its official endorsement from the Food and Drug Administration for the treatment of TIAs following the Canadian trial[3] (Chapter 2). In the circumstances, no alternative dose could be contemplated, even though a lower dose is now more frequently employed with more theoretical than proven justification. Although the rate of unwanted effects with aspirin is apparently dose-related, such a relationship is imperfect, as shown by examination of the side effects reported with different dosages in British trials[15,16] (Table 5.6). The UK-TIA trial[16] showed no difference between the protective effects of 1200 mg and 300 mg daily against disabling or fatal strokes and nonvascular deaths, but there was a non-significant increase in the rate of intracerebral hemorrhage with the higher dose, although the numbers

TABLE 5.6. Complications of ASA in three trials.

Study	TASS[4]	UK male MD[15]	UK TIA trial[16]	
ASA dose, mg	1300	500	300	1200
No. of patients	1527	3429	806	815
Discontinued, GI bleed	1.2%	2%	2/6%	4.7%
Hospitalized, GI bleed	1.0%	—	1.5%	2.3%
Indigestion, vomiting, etc.	41.1%	—	29.4%	38.8%

were very small. Aspirin produced some unwanted effects more frequently than did ticlopidine even in low dosage (Table 5.6).

At the initiation of CATS, there was no important evidence that aspirin was of value in the prevention of *recurrent* stroke. Subsequently the ESPS results[17] indicated that in a consortium of patients with cerebrovascular diseases, including 29% with moderate completed strokes, aspirin plus dipyridamole gave a 33% risk reduction. The AICLA study[18] included some patients with completed ischemic stroke benefitted from aspirin with a 40% risk reduction, although the population was not strictly comparable to that of CATS.

The benefit obtained with ticlopidine is presumably through preventing both platelet deposition upon exposed subintimal collagen and upon the further deposition of platelets upon each other at such sites, but this may not be the entire explanation of its mechanism. In the TIMAD study, a reduction in microaneurysm formation was shown in insulin-treated diabetic patients with retinopathy, for which both antiaggregating and antithrombotic effects in the retinal arterioles were considered to be responsible.[10]

Conclusion

In patients with atheromatous (or diabetic) vasculopathy, the antiplatelet agent ticlopidine can reduce the risk of further serious events such as strokes. In studies comparing it directly with aspirin, ticlopidine has afforded a significantly greater protective effect. The relationship of the enhanced protection conferred by ticlopidine to its broader mode of platelet inhibition is speculative. Frequency of unwanted effects of ticlopidine is slightly greater than that in patients taking aspirin, and the unwanted effects themselves are different, although risk of life-threatening complications is no greater than with aspirin and the risk-benefit ratio (comparing the number of permanent vascular events suffered with the risk of severe neutropenia) is firmly in favor of ticlopidine's use. Physicians using ticlopidine become comfortable with it, given the reassurance of strict monitoring in the first 3 months, when twice-weekly blood counts and vigilance for diarrhea or skin rashes are utilized. Probably in all patients, but especially in those who cannot take or have failed to respond to aspirin (whether due to its different mechanisms of platelet inhibition, to its effects in small vessels, or to both), ticlopidine appears to be a useful agent for prevention of secondary irreversible vascular events in patients shown to be at high risk.

References

1. Craven LL. Prevention of coronary and cerebral thrombosis. *Miss Valley Med J* 1952;**74**:213–215.
2. Craven LL. Experiences with aspirin (acetylsalicylic acid) in the nonspecific prophylaxis of coronary thrombosis. *Miss Valley Med J* 1956;**78**:38–44.
3. Canadian Cooperative Study Group. A randomized trial of aspirin and sulfinpyrazone in threatened stroke. *New Engl J Med* 1978;**299**:53–56.
4. Hass WK, Easton JD, Adams HP Jr. A randomized trial comparing ticlopidine hydrochloride with aspirin for the prevention of stroke in high-risk patients. *New Engl J Med* 1989;**321**:501–507.
5. Gent M, Blakely JD, et al. The Canadian American Ticlopidine Study (CATS) in thromboembolic stroke. *Lancet* 1989;1215–1220.
6. Gent M, Blakely JA, Hachinski VC, et al. A secondary prevention randomized trial of suloctidil in patients with a recent history of thromboembolic stroke. *Stroke* 1985;**16**:416–424.
7. Helmers C. High-dose acetylsalicylic acid after cerebral infarction. *Stroke* 1987;**18**:325–334.
8. Gent M, Blakely JA, Easton JD, et al. The Canadian American ticlopidine study in thrombotic stroke. Design, organization and baseline results. *Stroke* 1988;**19**:1203–1210.
9. Tohgi H. The Japanese ticlopidine study in transient ischemic attacks. *Sang Thrombose Vaisseaux* 1990;**2(4)**:19–22.
10. TIMAD study group. Ticlopidine treatment reduces the progression of nonproliferative diabetic retinopathy. *Arch Ophthalmol* 1990;**108**:1577–1583.
11. Uchiyama S, Osawa M, Maruyama M. Ticlopidine therapy in TIA and RIND (in Japanese). *Gendai No Shinyro* 1980;**22**:1325–1330.
12. Murakami G, Toyokura Y, Omae T, et al. Effects of aspirin and ticlopidine on transient ischemic attack (in Japanese). *Sindan To Chiryo* 1986;**74**:2255–2274.
13. Sato R, Uchiyama S, Nagayama T, et al. Recurrence and prophylaxis of ischemic cerebrovascular disorders in the aspect of platelet aggregation (in Japanese). *Neurol Therap* 1986;**3**:173–178.
14. Uchiyama S, Sone R, Nagayama T, et al. Combination therapy with low-dose aspirin and ticlopidine in cerebral ischemia. *Stroke* 1989;**20**:1643–1647.
15. Peta R, Gray R, Collins R, et al. Randomized trial of prophylactic daily aspirin in British male doctors. *Brit Med J* 1988;**296**:313–316.
16. UK-TIA Study Group. United Kingdom transient ischemic attack (UK-TIA) trial: interim results. *Brit Med J* 1988;**296**:316–319.
17. ESPS Group. European Stroke Prevention Study. *Stroke* 1990;**21**:1122–1130.
18. Bousser MG, Eschwege E, Haguenau M, et al. "AICLA" controlled trial of aspirin and dipyridamole in the secondary prevention of atherothrombotic cerebral ischemia. *Stroke* 1983;**14**:5–14.

6
Clinical Trials of Ticlopidine in Patients with Intermittent Claudication

Lars Janzon

Atherosclerosis—Main Cause in Peripheral Arterial Disease

Atherosclerosis is the main pathophysiologic process behind peripheral arterial disease (PAD).[1] Like other atherosclerotic manifestations, PAD is more common in old people than young and more common in men than women. The clinical spectrum of PAD ranges from an asymptomatic stage with weak leg arterial pulsations, a femoral bruit, or an abnormal systolic arm-ankle pressure gradient, to a symptomatic stage with intermittent claudication, rest pain, and gangrene. Depending on different clinical criteria and varying methods of assessing leg blood flow, the prevalence of PAD varies from one study to another. Several publications have presented prevalence estimates of intermittent claudication as being 2% in middle-aged men and 1% in middle-aged women.[2-4] Study findings by Reunanen et al.[2] support the clinical experience that PAD is becoming more common in women. Among 30–39-year-olds in that study, the prevalence of intermittent claudication was twice as high in women as in men.

The main risk factors associated with PAD are smoking, hypertension, hyperlipidemia, and diabetes.[5] Prevalence of these risk factors in patients with intermittent claudication has been assessed in several studies.[3-5] The common experience is that almost all patients are or have been smokers, about 30% of them have hypertension, 16% have hyperlipidemia, and 10% have diabetes. Many patients are exposed to more than one risk factor. In a study by Janzon et al., including 208 consecutive male patients 30–75 years of age, 18% of patients were smokers with hypertension and hyperlipidemia. The systolic arm-ankle pressure gradient, which can be considered to be a semiquantitative estimate of the amount of atherosclerosis in the main arteries from heart to ankle level, has been found to be linearly related to the number of risk factors.[6]

Intermittent Claudication—a Marker of Generalized Atherosclerotic Disease

About 25% of patients submitted for surgical evaluation are later operated on with reconstructive vascular surgery or angioplasty. Although surgery for many patients leads to a complete restoration of function, the incidence of reocclusions, especially following femoropopliteal bypasses, is high.[7] In the absence of surgery, disease progression is the rule. Strandness and Stahler[8] found that 52% of the patients progressed as determined by segmental systolic pressures and angiography. From the Framingham study it has been calculated that further occlusions can be expected in 40% of patients within 5 years.[9] The annual amputation rate varies in published studies depending on differences in patient age, stage of disease, and prevalence of diabetes, i.e. from less than 1% to 3%.[10,11] Diabetic patients have been found to have a higher amputation rate than non-diabetic patients.[12]

It is well documented that atherosclerosis is a disease afflicting the whole vascular tree, and that patients with peripheral artery disease have a high cardiovascular and cerebrovascular morbidity and mortality rate. Thirty to 50 percent of patients with newly-diagnosed peripheral artery disease have signs or symptoms of coronary ischemia.[2,9] In the Framingham study men who had or who developed intermittent claudication suffered an annual mortality that averaged 39/1000 as compared to 10/1000 in men free of the affliction.[9] Similar results have been reported by Reunanen[2] and Källerö.[13]

Rationale for Antithrombotic Treatment

Clinical and preventive benefits associated with treatment of high blood pressure and hyperlipidemia as well as cessation of smoking have been evaluated in several studies.[14-16] No control trials have been performed to assess if and how the natural course in PAD can be improved by adequate treatment of known cardiovascular risk factors. In STIMS,[17] the Swedish Ticlopidine Multicentre Study, in which all smokers were given help and advice to quit smoking and all those with hypertension and hyperlipidemia received appropriate treatment, the incidence of myocardial infarction, stroke, and TIA in the placebo-treated control group remained at almost 30% during a mean 5.6-year observation period. The conclusion was that a treatment program including smoking counselling together with treatment of high blood pressure and hyperlipidemia still seems to be "too little too late." The antithrombotic treatment role in patients with PAD should be considered with these facts in mind.

Ticlopidine's efficacy in preventing myocardial infarction, stroke, and leg blood flow impairment necessitating vascular surgery or amputation has been evaluated in a number of placebo-control trials. However, many of these studies have had too limited statistical power to document beneficial effects associated with treatment because of small cohorts and short study durations.

In 1982 in the *Journal of Clinical Pathology*,[18] Aukland et al. reported the results from a placebo-controlled trial of ticlopidine in 65 male outpatients with stable intermittent claudication. After a placebo run-in period of 4 weeks, patients were randomly allocated to treatment with ticlopidine or placebo, 250 mg twice daily for 12 months. No presentation was given of expected treatment effect or expected statistical power. Outcomes assessment included follow-up of resting pressure index, claudication distance, maximum walking distance, and calf blood flow at rest and during reactive hyperemia. The publication did not include any presentation of outcome in the placebo-treated group. In the ticlopidine group there was a small but statistically insignificant increase in calf peak flow. Other parameters used in the evaluation remained unchanged.

Stiegler et al. reported in 1984[19] on the results from a placebo-controlled study of ticlopidine in 43 patients with intermittent claudication. Serial angiography of the lower limbs was used to assess ticlopidine's efficacy in preventing progression of obliterative arterial disease. The study was originally designed to include 240 patients, but recruitment was terminated early because of the occurrence of one case with erythroleukemia.

Patients were randomly allocated to treatment with ticlopidine and placebo, 250 mg twice daily. The distribution of known cardiovascular risk factors was similar in the two groups at baseline. Mean progression, as assessed by angiographic score, was 4.2 in the placebo group and 0.1 in the ticlopidine group, $p < 0.01$. It should be noted, however, that mean angiographic score at baseline was higher in the placebo group (24.9) than in the ticlopidine group (21.6).

Arcan et al. (1988, *Angiology*) reported the results from a French multicenter study designed to assess ticlopidine's effects on symptoms of intermittent claudication and prevention of ischemic thrombotic complications.[20] The study included 169 patients who had suffered from intermittent claudication for at least 12 months and who had a treadmill walking distance of between 50 and 300 meters. Existence of obstructive arterial disease was confirmed by either angiography or by doppler studies. After a 4-week, single-blind placebo run-in period, patients were randomly allocated to placebo or ticlopidine, 250 mg twice daily. Patients were examined every 4 weeks with treadmill testing of walking distance.

The treatment outcome was decided by an independent validation committee. Success was defined as absence of cardiovascular events, improvement of treadmill walking distance (i.e., an increase greater than 50% with respect to baseline at final evaluation and at least two of three previous visits), and functional improvement as assessed by both patient and investigator.

This study was designed to have 90% power at 5% significance level to detect a 50% success rate in the ticlopidine group as compared to 30% in the placebo group. Final evaluation was performed on the "intent-to-treat" basis. Distribution

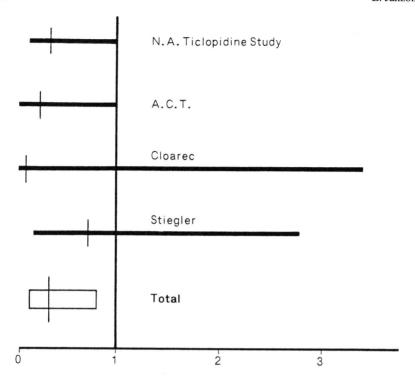

FIGURE 6.1. Metaanalysis of ticlopidine's treatment effect in patients with obliterative arterial disease. Source: *Thromb Haemost* 1989;**62(2)**:681–685.

of age, sex, and cardiovascular risk factors as well as severity of disease were similar in the two groups at randomization.

After 6 months, the treatment success rate was 44.5% in the ticlopidine group and 34.8% in the placebo group. This difference was not statistically significant. The mean increase in walking distance, however, was significantly greater in the ticlopidine group than in the placebo group. The mean increase in pain-free walking distance, baseline vs. final follow-up, was 194 meters in the ticlopidine group and 124 meters in the placebo group (p = 0.03). Total walking distance, baseline vs. follow-up, increased with a mean 236 meters in the ticlopidine group and 170 meters in the placebo group (p = 0.04).

No data were presented on the development of arm-ankle pressure ratios in relation to change in walking distance. Furthermore, no accounting was offered for potential effects of other treatment, such as antihypertensive medications, lipid-lowering drugs, or antismoking counseling. In both groups 36% were current smokers. Of the 12 cases suffering cerebrovascular or peripheral ischemic episodes, only 2 in the ticlopidine group required vascular surgical treatment (p = 0.03).

Two other control trials of ticlopidine in patients with intermittent claudication have presented reports in abstract publications of the drug's beneficial

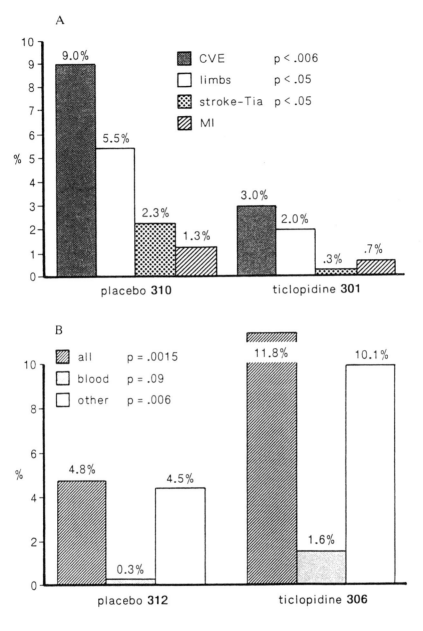

FIGURE 6.2. Effects of ticlopidine on incidence of cardiovascular events in patients with intermittent claudication. Source: *Thromb Haemost* 1989;**62(2)**:681–685.

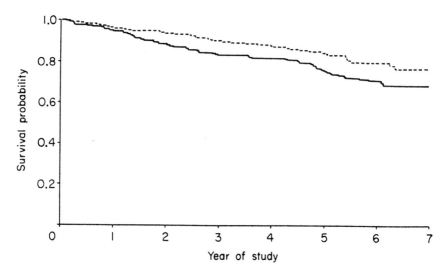

FIGURE 6.3. STIMS on-treatment analysis of ticlopidine's effects on incidence of acute MI, stroke and TIA in patients with intermittent claudication. Log-rank test for treatment difference: p = 0.017. (- - - -) = ticlopidine, (—) = placebo. Source: *J Intern Med* 1990;**227**:301–308.

effects on walking performance in patients with PAD.[21,22] Studies have also been published indicating that ticlopidine treatment improves healing of ischemic leg ulcers.[23]

Meta-analysis of four of the above-mentioned, placebo-controlled trials of ticlopidine in patients with peripheral arterial disease reported by Boissel et al.[24] revealed that ticlopidine treatment was associated with a significantly lower incidence of cardiovascular events (3%) as compared to placebo treatment (9%). The analysis included 611 patients with treatment periods varying from 6 to 12 months. Walking impairment, sex distribution, and prevalence of hyperlipidemia were similar in the two groups at randomization. Similar treatment effects were observed for all individual endpoints, i.e., myocardial infarction, stroke/TIA, and vascular surgery.

The incidence of side effects was 11.8% in the ticlopidine group and 4.8% in the placebo group. Hematological side effects (in each case granulocytopenia) were 1.6% in the ticlopidine group and 0.3% in the placebo group. Blood counts returned to normal after withdrawal from study treatment.

The question of whether ticlopidine can reduce the high cardio- and cerebrovascular morbidity and mortality rates in claudicants was again addressed in STIMS, the Swedish Ticlopidine Multicentre Study.[17] Included in the trial were 687 patients younger than 70 years of age with intermittent claudication as defined by the WHO questionnaire. Presence of leg artery occlusive disease was

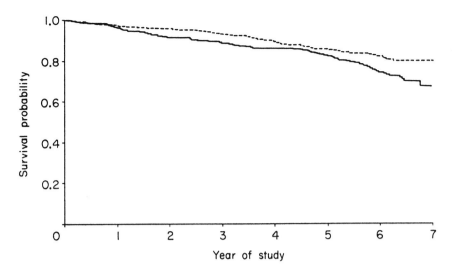

FIGURE 6.4. Intention-to-treat analysis of total mortality, including all deaths until the end of the trial. Log-rank test for treatment difference: p = 0.015. (———) = ticlopidine, (——) = placebo. Source: *J Intern Med* 1990;**227**:301–308

confirmed by an abnormal systolic pressure gradient between the upper arm and the ankle.

About 50% of the patients had had intermittent claudication for more than 3 years. Prior to entry, 30% had undergone reconstructive vascular surgery. One of five (20%) had a history of myocardial infarction, 2–3% had suffered a stroke, 95% were or had been smokers. Thirty percent had serum cholesterol values exceeding 6.3 mmol, and half had a systolic blood pressure above 160 mmHg. All patients were monitored for known cardiovascular risk factors and received other interventions if necessary. The effect of cigarette smoking on the progress of atherosclerosis was explained, and all patients were encouraged to abstain from smoking. Patients were followed up every 3 months. The study was designed to have 90% power at 5% significance level to detect a 50% reduction in incidence of the compound endpoint: myocardial infarction, stroke, and TIA.

All patients were identified for evaluation of status at the end of the trial. Median duration of observation, from entry to final evaluation or to an endpoint and/or death if earlier, was 5.6 years. Completing the study were 146 of the 340 placebo-treated patients and 120 of the 346 ticlopidine patients. Those withdrawn from the study because of adverse events, intercurrent disease, or other reasons included 195 in the placebo group and 226 in the ticlopidine group. At the trial's end there were 89 deaths in the placebo group and 64 in the ticlopidine group. The 29% lower mortality rate in the ticlopidine group (p = 0.015) was entirely

TABLE 6.1. Effects of ticlopidine on mortality in patients with intermittent claudication: comparison of total and cause-specific mortality.

Underlying cause of death[1]	Placebo ($n = 341$)		Ticlopidine ($n = 346$)	
	n	%	n	%
Ischemic heart disease 410–414	54 (12)[2]	15.8	31 (9)[2]	9.0
Cerebrovascular disease 430–438	4 (1)	1.2	5 (3)	1.4
Cancer 140–239	15 (1)	4.4	17 (3)	4.9
Other	16 (9)	4.7	11 (2)	3.2
Total	89[3] (23)	26.1	64[3] (17)	18.5

[1] According to ICD code, 8th revised version.
[2] Figures in parentheses denote deaths which occurred following a nonfatal endpoint.
[3] Statistically significant at $P = 0.015$.
Source: *J Intern Med* 1990;**227**:301–308.

explained by the lower number of deaths from myocardial infarction, 31 vs. 54. Other causes of death were similar in the two groups.

The incidence of myocardial infarction, stroke, and TIA in patients on treatment (excluding events that occurred more than 15 days after discontinuation of treatment because of side effects or because of intercurrent disease) was 13.8% in the ticlopidine group and 22.4% in the placebo group (p = 0.017). When time for observation was taken into account, the corresponding risk ratio was 0.66 (95% confidence interval, 0.45–0.96).

The frequency of side effects was greater in the ticlopidine group than in the placebo group, with 26 placebo patients and 73 ticlopidine patients being withdrawn from treatment permanently due to side effects. Diarrhea was the most frequently reported side effect. Hematological side effects (i.e., thrombocytopenia, leukopenia, or pancytopenia) were reported for 7 patients, 2% in the ticlopidine group and none in the placebo group. The clinical course was benign in this group after drug discontinuation.

At two participating clinics in STIMS, follow-up also included an evaluation of systolic arm-ankle pressure gradient after 1 year of treatment. Separate analyses were made for the best and worst leg, i.e., leg with greatest and smallest pressure difference at entry. After 1 year of treatment there was a significantly

TABLE 6.2. Change in systolic arm/ankle pressure gradient after 1 year of treatment.

Arm-ankle pressure gradient: baseline value vs. 1 year follow-up	Worst leg		Best leg	
	Placebo %	Ticlopidine %	Placebo %	Ticlopidine %
Deterioration	17.6	10.3[1]	29.7	16.7[1]
Unchanged	63.7	66.2	56.7	63.2
Improvement	18.6	23.5	13.7	20.1
Baseline value X ± SD	53 ± 26	50 ± 23	26 ± 28	26 ± 26

[1] p < 0.05.

smaller percentage (p = 0.05) of deteriorations (more than 15 mmHg increase of arm-ankle pressure gradient) in the ticlopidine-treated group. The greater percentage of improvements (>15 mmHg reduction of the arm-ankle pressure difference) in the ticlopidine group was not statistically significant.

Conclusion

Several studies have documented the health benefits associated with cessation of smoking and with treatment of hypertension and hyperlipidemia.[14-16] Although we lack data from control trials, it seems fair to assume that progression of disease in patients with intermittent claudication can be slowed by treatment of these known atherosclerotic risk factors. However, considering the thrombotic event underlying the most and common and most serious vascular complication in patients with PAD, i.e., acute myocardial infarction, it does not seem rational to concentrate only on a therapeutic approach that can be supposed to influence only the development of atherosclerosis. Platelet antiaggregatory agents may, therefore, be considered the most important part of a treatment program for patients with peripheral arterial disease known to be at high risk of myocardial infarction, ischemic stroke, and vascular death.

References

1. Strandness DE Jr. *Peripheral Arterial Disease*. Boston, Little Brown, 1969.
2. Reunanen A, Takkunen H, Aromaa A. Prevalence of intermittent claudication and its effect on mortality. *Acta Med Scand* 1982;**211**:249–256.
3. Hughson WG, Mann J, Garrod A. Intermittent claudication: prevalence and risk factors. *Br Med J* 1978;**1**:1379–1381.
4. Isacsson S-O. Venous occlusion plethysmography in 55-year-old men. A population study in Malmö, Sweden (thesis). *Acta Med Scand* 1972;**191**:537.
5. Gordon T, Kannel WB. Predisposition to atherosclerosis in the head, heart and legs. The Framingham study. *JAMA* 1972;**221**:661–666.
6. Janzon L, Bergentz S-E, Ericsson BF, Lindell SE. The arm-ankle pressure gradient in relation to cardiovascular risk factors in intermittent claudication. *Circulation* 1981;**63(6)**:1339–1341.
7. Ruckley CV. Claudication. *Br Med J* 1986;**292**:970–971.
8. Strandness D Jr, Stahler C. Arteriosclerosis obliterans. *JAMA* 1966;**196**:1–4.
9. Kannel WB, Shurtleff D. The natural history of arteriosclerosis obliterans. *Cardiovasc Clin* 1971;**37**:3.
10. Tillgren C. Obliterative disease of the lower limbs. II. A study of the cause of the disease. *Acta Med Scand* 1965;**178**:103.
11. Silbert S, Zazeela H. Prognosis in arteriosclerotic peripheral vascular disease. *JAMA* 1958;**166**:186.
12. Boyd AM. The natural course of arteriosclerosis of the lower extremities. *Proc Roy Soc Med* 1962;**55**:591.

13. Källerö KS. Mortality and morbidity in patients with intermittent claudication as defined by venous occlusion plethysmography. A ten year follow-up study. *J Chronic Dis* 1981;**34**:455–462.
14. Wilhelmsson C, Vedin JA, Elmfeldt D, Tibblin G, Whilhelmsen L. Smoking and myocardial infarction. *Lancet* 1975;**1**:415.
15. Hypertension Detection and Follow-up Program Cooperative Group. Five-year findings of the hypertension detection and follow-up program. I. Reduction in mortality of persons with high blood pressure, including mild hypertension. *JAMA* 1979;**242**:2562.
16. Coronary Heart Disease—Lipid Research Clinics Program. The lipid research clinics coronary primary prevention trial results. I. Reduction in incidence of coronary heart disease. II. The relationship of reduction in incidence of coronary heart disease to cholesterol lowering. *JAMA* 1984;**251**:351–374.
17. Janzon L, Bergqvist D, Boberg J, et al. Prevention of myocardial infarction and stroke in patients with intermittent claudication; effects of ticlopidine. Results from STIMS, the Swedish Ticlopidine Multicentre Study. *J Intern Med* 1990;**227**:301–308.
18. Aukland A, Hurlow RA, George AJ, Stuart J. Platelet inhibition with ticlopidine in atherosclerotic intermittent claudication. *J Clin Pathol* 1982;**35**:740–743.
19. Stiegler H, Hess H, Mietaschk A, Trampisch H-J, Ingrisch H. Einfluss von Ticlopidin auf die periphere obliterierende arteriopathie. *Dtsch Med Wschr* 1984;**109**:1240–1243.
20. Arcan JC, Blanchard JF, Boissel JP, Destors JM, Panak EA. Multicenter double-blind study of ticlopidine in the treatment of intermittent claudication and the prevention of its complications. *Angiology* 1988;**39(9)**:802–811.
21. Ellis DJ. Treatment of intermittent claudication with ticlopidine. Abstract addendum. International Committee on Thrombosis and Haemostasis 32nd Annual Meeting and the Mediterranean League Against Thromboembolic Diseases, 9th Congress. Jerusalem, June 1–6, 1986.
22. Cloarec M, Caillard PH, Mouren X. Double-blind clinical trial of ticlopidine versus placebo in peripheral atherosclerotic disease of the legs. *Thromb Res* 1986;(suppl 6):160.
23. Katsumara T, Mishima Y, Kamiya K, Sakaguchi S, Tanabe T, Sakuma A. Therapeutic effect of ticlopidine, a new inhibitor of platelet aggregation, on chronic arterial occlusive diseases, a double-blind study versus placebo. *Angiology* 1982;**33(6)**:357–367.
24. Boissel JP, Peyrieux JC, Destors JM. Is it possible to reduce the risk of cardiovascular events in subjects suffering from intermittent claudication of the lower limbs? *Thromb Heamost* 1989;**62(2)**:681–685.

7
Clinical Trials of Ticlopidine in Patients with Coronary Artery Disease

Francesco Balsano and Francesco Violi

Acute coronary syndromes, including myocardial infarction, unstable angina, and early complications occurring after aortocoronary bypass or angioplasty, are well recognized conditions in which *in situ* activation of platelets and the coagulation cascade play a pivotal role. Therefore, anticoagulant or antiplatelet drugs have been employed to reduce vascular thrombosis and minimize clinical complications secondary to vascular occlusion. In regard to antiplatelet drugs, many studies have been performed with aspirin, an inhibitor of the cyclooxygenase enzyme that prevents formation of thromboxane TXA_2, a potent aggregating and vasoconstrictor agent.

Most of these studies have documented aspirin's beneficial effect. In patients with suspected acute myocardial infarction (MI), 160 mg/day of aspirin have been shown to significantly reduce vascular death and reinfarction.[1] A significant reduction of vascular death or fatal or nonfatal MI was obtained when patients with unstable angina were given 324–1300 mg/day of aspirin.[1] Aspirin has also been administered to patients who survived the acute phase of MI in order to evaluate its capability for reducing late vascular death and reinfarction. However, most of these studies produced equivocal results, suggesting that the effect of antiplatelet in this stage of coronary heart disease needs further investigation.[1] Aspirin's effect in the acute or late occlusion of aortocoronary bypass has been extensively studied and has shown a reduction of bypass closure when the drug was administered as early as 24–48 hours after surgery. Finally, some preliminary reports suggest aspirin's usefulness in treating acute complications of coronary angioplasty.[1]

Many investigations have been planned on the basis of these beneficial effects of antiplatelet therapy in clinical models of coronary artery disease complicated by thrombosis in order to verify whether ticlopidine, an antiplatelet drug with a novel mechanism of action could be effective in reducing vascular complication occurring in the clinical situations reported above.

Ticlopidine has been employed in patients with unstable angina, aortocoronary bypass, or angioplasty but has never been systematically administered to patients with (MI). This chapter will analyze both the beneficial and unwanted effects of ticlopidine given to patients with coronary heart disease (CHD).

Unstable Angina

The term unstable angina is applied to various clinical conditions characterized by the "instability" of the coronary atherosclerotic process (see Chapter 1). Such instability is largely due to dynamic obstruction of the coronary tree superimposed on organic stenosis.[2] *In situ* platelet and coagulation activation are responsible for a "dynamic" thrombotic process potentially leading to complete vascular occlusion.[3] This explains why unstable angina is considered a potentially life-threatening coronary arterial syndrome, since in about 10–14% of cases it is complicated by vascular death and MI.[4]

As the result of differing clinical symptoms which have largely been considered under the term unstable angina, Braunwald[5] recently proposed a classification of this acute coronary arterial syndrome that takes into account: 1) the varying severity of its presentation—whether the onset is at rest and whether it has been present within the last 48 hours; 2) the clinical circumstances that accompany it, in particular, whether the angina is secondary to an extracardiac cause leading to an increased oxygen demand by the myocardium (as in fever, anemia, or tachyarrhythmia), or whether it is primarily due to accentuation of coronary ischemia or is postinfarctual, with an onset within the 2 weeks that follow a myocardial infarction; and 3) the presence or absence of transitory electrocardiographic abnormalities of the ST-T segment. Moreover, Braunwald suggested the usefulness of classifying patients on the basis of their therapeutic needs: 1) unstable angina occurring in the absence of, or during, minimal antianginal therapy; 2) unstable angina still present in spite of a correct therapy for a chronic and stable form; and 3) unstable angina refractory to maximal antianginal therapy with calcium antagonists + beta blockers + long-lasting nitrates.

Although an uncertain classification is still a characteristic of unstable angina, most studies of coronary artery morphology and biochemical markers have focused on the important role of platelets on the clinical evolution of unstable angina. This suggestion has been definitively confirmed by clinical trials with the platelet inhibitors, aspirin and ticlopidine.

Pathophysiology

The thrombotic complication of the coronary atherosclerotic plaque is the physiopathologic mechanism that determines onset of unstable angina. It generally occurs on an area of coronary stenosis, which may be complicated by ulceration or fissuration, thus leading to platelet and coagulation cascade activation.

It is the onset of such atherosclerotic complications, *not* the severity of coronary arterial lesion, that differentiates patients with stable or unstable angina. Thus, patients with stable or unstable angina have the same entity of coronary stenosis.[6] However, when sequential angiographic studies are performed before and after the appearance of instability, a progression of coronary artery stenosis may be observed, indicating that a dynamic process occurs during the progression from the stable to the unstable phase.[7-9]

Progression of stenosis severity is due mainly to intraplaque hemorrhage secondary to fissuring.[10] This process usually does not lead to vascular occlusion; instead it induces a major increase in severity of the lesion. It is probably a consequence of repeated atherosclerotic plaque alterations, as indicated by Falk's study[3] which demonstrated that 81% of coronary arterial thrombi are composed of a layered structure of different ages. These suggest that the progression of stenosis is due to repeated mural thrombi which may lead to complete vascular occlusion. These morphological studies have subsequently been confirmed by angioscopic studies performed by Sherman et al. on 10 patients with stable angina and 10 patients with unstable angina, the latter being defined as accelerated or at-rest angina.[11] It is noteworthy that all the patients with crescendo angina were shown to have complicated plaque in their coronary arteries. Further, coronary thrombus was detected in all the patients with at-rest angina. In contrast, none of the atherosclerotic lesions in patients with stable angina are of this type.

The crucial importance of coronary artery thrombosis detection early in the acute phase of unstable angina must be related to the "instability" of the thrombus which, in fact, undergoes rapid and intermittent fragmentation in 73% of cases and probably causes microembolization to the small intramyocardial arteries.[3]

This phenomenon, which is probably the cause of microinfarcts, is typical of unstable angina. Davies et al.[12] found intramyocardial platelet emboli in 44.4% of patients with unstable angina. It was seen in only 20.4% of patients who did not manifest this syndrome. These observations suggested that study of platelet function in unstable angina might further define the pathophysiology of myocardial ischemia. Fitzgerald et al.[13] studied the behavior of two stable platelet metabolites of TXA_2, 2-3 dinor-TXB_2, in urine and plasma levels of 11-dehydro-TXB_2 in 16 patients with unstable angina and in patients with stable angina. They found an increase of both of these indices of *in vivo* platelet activation in 84% of pain episodes in patients with at-rest angina; but not in patients with stable coronary disease, both at rest and after exercise. It is noteworthy that in 50% of patients with increased formation of TXA_2 metabolites, no angina episodes were recorded, suggesting that this elevation could be related to silent ischemia. This suggested that episodes of symptomatic and asymptomatic vasospasm could be related to the platelets' release of vasoconstrictor substances such as TXA_2.

This hypothesis has been verified in a subsequent study by Vejar et al.,[14] who studied 21 patients with at-rest angina or deterioration of stable angina. Patients with unstable angina were characterized by episodic increases in the urinary excretion of 11-dehydro-TXA_2, further supporting the concept that platelet activation occurs in this kind of coronary disease. However, a direct relation between myocardial ischemia and platelet activation could not be proved. Eleven out of 21 episodes of myocardial ischemia were not accompanied by increased urinary excretion of 11-dehydro-TXB_2. In addition, only three episodes of enhanced 11-dehydro-TXB$_2$ excretion were associated with ST-segment changes. A frequent association between increased excretion of 11-dehydro-TXB$_2$ and myocardial ischemia was observed only in the case of chest pain with ST segment changes. Finally, increased excretion of 11-dehydro-TXB$_2$ was also recorded in patients who had been given aspirin, and in these cases also, this increase was not always accompanied by ST-segment changes. This last finding was in accordance with two previous clinical trials in which aspirin administration was unable to modify incidence and severity of myocardial ischemia[15,16].

When considered together, these studies exploring the behavior of TXA$_2$ metabolites in patients with unstable angina strongly suggest that platelet activation is a frequent feature of this coronary syndrome. A clear-cut association, however, between increased formation of TXA$_2$ and myocardial ischemia could not be proved, suggesting that other mechanisms or that platelet metabolites contribute to modification of vascular tone.

Histological, angiographic, and biochemical studies have stressed the role that platelets play in the dynamic process leading to unstable angina, which is the basis for the extensive number of clinical trials with antiplatelet drugs in which the aim was to evaluate if such therapy could modify the clinical course of unstable angina.

Antiplatelet Drugs for Unstable Angina

Three drugs that inhibit platelet function, i.e., aspirin, sulfinpyrazone, and ticlopidine, have been used in unstable angina to prevent cardiovascular complications. Aspirin irreversibly acetylates cyclooxygenase enzyme, thus preventing the formation of thromboxane A2 (TXA$_2$) a potent aggregating and vaso-constrictor agent. At a daily dosage of 160 to 300 mg, aspirin reduces platelet TXA$_2$ formation by more than 90%.[17] Sulfinpyrazone has been shown to prolong platelet survival. This effect seems to be related to inhibition of the cyclooxy-genase pathway.[17] Sulfinpyrazone is usually given at a dose of 800 mg/day. Ticlopidine is a new antiplatelet drug that inhibits ADP-mediated platelet aggregation and prevents fibrinogen binding to the platelet membrane.[18,19] Ticlopidine's antiplatelet effect appears 24 to 48 hours after administering a daily dose of 500 mg, which indicates that inhibition of platelet function is due to active metabolites.[20]

Five trials using drugs that inhibit platelet function have been carried out in patients with unstable angina. In the first two studies,[15,16] the active drug was aspirin given at the dosage of 324–1300 mg/day (Table 7.1). In two other trials[21,22] aspirin at low or high dosage was compared with heparin given intravenously. In the second trial[23] the active drug was ticlopidine. Although an overall analysis of the trials indicated the clinical efficacy of therapy with platelet inhibitors, the different methodological approaches used should be evaluated to clarify the findings.

TABLE 7.1. Effect of antiplatelet therapy on vascular death and myocardial infarction in patients with unstable angina.

	Study design	Therapy	Follow-up	Risk reduction
Lewis et al.	Randomized	Placebo	12 weeks	51% p = 0.0002
	Double blind	ASA		
Cairns et al.	Randomized	Placebo	24 months	30% p = 0.072
	Double blind	ASA		
Theroux et al.	Randomized	Placebo	7 days	
	Double blind	ASA		72% p = 0.01
		Heparin		93% p = 0.009
Balsano et al.	Randomized	Standard therapy	3 months	
		Standard therapy + ticlopidine		46.3% p = 0.009
RISC	Randomized	Placebo	90 days	
	Double blind	ASA		62% p = 0.0001
		Heparin		5% n.s.

There were some differences in methodological approaches adopted in the American and Canadian studies in which aspirin was the active drug (Table 7.1). The American study[15] included patients within 48 hours of symptom onset, whereas the Canadian Study[16] randomized patients within 198 hours from hospitalization. Since the clinical course of patients with unstable angina is quickly complicated by serious cardiovascular accidents, the delayed inclusion of patients in the Canadian Study could have reduced the apparent efficacy of aspirin.

In addition, the Canadian study follow-up duration was 24 months, although the clinical complications of unstable angina usually occur in the first 1–3 months. Evaluation of the results by intention-to-treat analysis revealed that in the American study aspirin significantly reduced risk of fatal and nonfatal myocardial infarction by 55%, whereas vascular death was reduced by 51%, an insignificant difference. Conversely, the Canadian study showed that aspirin was able to reduce vascular death by 42%, whereas myocardial infarction was not significantly influenced. Finally, sulfinpyrazone was found to be ineffective and was analyzed as a placebo. In the American study adverse reactions and side effects, including epigastric burning and discomfort, decreased hemoglobin concentration, or occult blood in the stool, were equally distributed between the two treatment groups. Discontinuation of treatment because of side effects was 1.4% in both the aspirin and placebo groups.

In the Canadian study side effects (probably due to medication) occurred in 44% of patients. Gastrointestinal disturbances, including peptic ulcer and melena, were subsequently observed in patients taking aspirin. These side effects were 29% more common in patients given aspirin than in those given the other medications (p = 0.014). In addition, about 27% of patients taking aspirin withdrew from the study, 10% of these because of side effects.

Theroux et al.[21] compared aspirin at a dosage of 600 mg/day with heparin (1000 U/h) given intravenously until discharge, which usually occurred after a week. They included patients with at-rest angina occurring within 24 hours prior to the time of randomization. Myocardial infarction, refractory angina, and vascular death were analyzed. The study showed that both aspirin and heparin were able to reduce nonfatal myocardial infarction, whereas refractory angina was reduced only by heparin. There were no additive effects in patients given both aspirin and heparin. It is noteworthy that vascular death was not observed, and myocardial infarction was diagnosed 36 ± 30 hours after randomization, which suggests that, at least in this type of unstable angina, occurrence of myocardial infarction is premature.

Complications and side effects had a low frequency, with 9% of patients taking aspirin and 9.3% of patients taking the placebo experiencing gastrointestinal disturbances or bleeding. The latter was relatively more frequent in patients taking heparin. Frequency of study discontinuation was very low in the aspirin (1.6%), heparin (5%), and placebo (2.5%) groups.

The RISC study[22] included patients with unstable angina or non-Q-wave myocardial infarction treated with low doses of aspirin (75 mg) or heparin given intravenously at a dosage of 5000 U every 6 hours during the first 24 hours followed by 3750 U every 6 hours in the following 4 days. This study demonstrated aspirin's protective effect against myocardial infarction and death, and the fact that heparin was ineffective. No further benefit was derived from simultaneous administration of aspirin and heparin. Heparin's lack of beneficial effect in this study is at variance with the results of Theroux et al. However, in the RISC study, heparin was given by intermittent infusion, and 81% of the patients were treated 24 hours after admission.

This study also showed relatively infrequent side effects, which were most often characterized by gastrointestinal disturbances. Only 18% of patients taking aspirin and 1.3% of patients taking placebo discontinued treatment.

In view of the results of the four studies, it is apparent that aspirin has protective effects against ischemic episodes occurring after symptom onset. Low doses of aspirin were effective and enjoyed a lower incidence of side effects. Anticoagulant therapy with heparin, given by continuous infusion, seems to be very effective in patients at high risk, such as those with at-rest angina, whereas it appears to be ineffective when given to patients with other clinical syndromes.

Efficacy of antiplatelet drugs in unstable angina has also been analyzed using ticlopidine. Following the same methodological approach used in the American study but including males and females, Balsano et al.[23] treated unstable angina patients with a standard therapy or a standard therapy plus ticlopidine (250 mg twice a day).

After 3–6 months of follow-up, the study showed a significant *reduction* in vascular death and nonfatal myocardial infarction by 46.3%, and in fatal and nonfatal myocardial infarction by 53.2%. The effect appeared after 15 days of treatment and was most evident in patients with a previous history of myocardial infarction. Side effects observed in the group taking ticlopidine were most frequently gastrointestinal disturbances (9.7%) and skin rash (1.9%). Fifteen patients (4.9%) taking ticlopidine discontinued treatment, 10 for gastrointestinal discomfort, and five for skin reactions.

These findings support the key role played by platelets in the clinical evolution of unstable angina. Comparison of risk reduction obtained with aspirin or ticlopidine clearly shows that both drugs can reduce the occurrence of serious vascular complications by about 50%. Comparison between these two drugs is necessary in order to assess their risk/benefit in unstable angina patients.

Conclusion

On the basis of results observed in clinical trials, the use of antiplatelet drugs in patients with unstable angina is to be recommended. In the case of high-risk patients, such as those with at-rest angina, anticoagulant therapy with continuous intravenous infusion of heparin could be started immediately and followed after 1 week by aspirin or ticlopidine. Since there are no laboratory tests to definitely support diagnosis of unstable angina, patients to be treated should include those with typical symptoms of chest pains and ECG alterations. They should be treated as soon as possible, preferably within 24 hours of hospitalization, to avoid the early occurrence of myocardial infarction.

Aortocoronary Bypass

One of the most important clinical problems related to evolution of aortocoronary bypass is its early and late occlusion. Early occlusion usually occurs between 1 and 6 months after operation. Its frequency is, to a certain extent, quite variable depending on several risk factors that may increase risk of bypass closure. Low blood flow of vein graft, vein damage during operation, dislipidemia, and a smoking habit are factors that increase risk of occlusion.[24] Bypass closure is about 18–25% during the first 6 months, thereafter it tends to decrease.[25]

Physiopathology

Early occlusion is due to a thrombotic process occurring on damaged endothelium. This leads to platelet deposition, thrombus formation, and vein graft occlusion. This phenomenon is quite evident a few hours after vein graft insertion. In an experimental model Iosa et al.[26] showed that as early as 2 hours after operation endothelium was lost; furthermore, 94% of the grafts showed inflammation, hemorrhage, and necrosis. At this stage thrombotic phenomena already have occurred. These may induce graft closure just 24 hours after operation.

Late vein graft occlusion resembles vascular occlusion occurring on the atherosclerotic lesion. In fact, within 1 year of operation, a proliferation of smooth muscle cells may occur.[27] Further vascular lesions include *de novo* synthesis of connective tissue and lipid accumulation, with a progressive reduction of vascular lumen.[28] The physiopathologic mechanism leading to late occlusion has not been completely clarified, but it is likely that platelet aggregation and adhesion to the damaged endothelium promote intimal changes occurring at this stage after vein graft lesion.[28]

On this physiopathologic basis, antiplatelet therapy has been utilized in order to reduce early and late occlusion and, in fact, antiplatelet treatment with aspirin, dipyridamole, or sulfinpyrazone have proved to be effective in reducing graft closure. This effect is more evident when treatment takes place as early as 24 hours after operation. Further delay of antiplatelet treatment did not seem to be efficacious.[28]

Clinical Trials with Ticlopidine

Ticlopidine has been preliminarily given to mongrel dogs in order to assess its capacity to inhibit graft occlusion. When administered up to 6 weeks after implantation of arterial dacron grafts, ticlopidine increased their patency rate.[29]

Ticlopidine treatment has been given in three different trials where it was compared to placebo or anticoagulant drug.

Chevigné et al.[30] studied 77 patients who had undergone aortocoronary bypass. The study design was randomized, double-blind, placebo-controlled (Table 7.2). Patients were given placebo or ticlopidine (250 mg bid) and monitored for 3 months. The study endpoint was graft occlusion, which was examined by thallium myocardial scintigraphy and angiography. Analysis of graft patency (graft-by-graft) by the intention-to-treat method showed no significant difference between ticlopidine and placebo (10.1% occlusion in ticlopidine group vs. 20.3% in placebo group). On the other hand, analysis on treatment showed a significant reduction of graft occlusion in the ticlopidine group (7.1% in the ticlopidine group vs. 21.8% in the placebo group; p < 0.02). Similar findings were observed through analysis of graft patency (patient-by-patient). While analysis by intention-to-treat did not show significant differences between the two groups, analysis on treatment indicated that ticlopidine significantly reduces bypass closure.

During treatment few side effects were noted. In the ticlopidine group, two patients suffered from bleeding complications, and three complained of gastrointestinal disturbances. Serial hematological examination, conducted up to 90 days, did not show particular changes in either the ticlopidine or placebo groups.

Rothlin et al.[31] compared ticlopidine and an oral anticoagulant in a randomized unblinded study. They administered ticlopidine (250 mg bid) or acenocoumarol to 166 patients who had undergone aortocoronary bypass 24 hours before and 24–48 hours before, respectively. Patients were followed up for 3 months, then an angiographic examination was performed to evaluate vein graft patency (Table 7.1).

Prothrombin activity of patients taking acenocoumarol was 20–25%. Seventy-eight of 83 patients in the ticlopidine group and 71 of 83 patients in the acenocoumarol group completed the study with postoperative coronary angiography. The ticlopidine group had 43% of its patients with at least one

TABLE 7.2. Ticlopidine on the prevention of aortocoronary bypass closure.

	Study design	Follow-up	Treatment	Bypass closure
Chevigné et al.	Randomized Double blind	3 months	Placebo Ticlopidine	21.8% 7.1% $p < 0.02$ [1]
Rothlin et al.	Randomized	3 months	Acenocoumarol Ticlopidine	42% 43%
		10 days	Placebo Ticlopidine	13.4% 7.1% $p < 0.05$
Limet et al.	Randomized Double blind	6 months	Placebo Ticlopidine	24% 15% $p < 0.02$
		1 year	Placebo Ticlopidine	26% 15% $p < 0.01$

[1] On-treatment analysis.

occluded graft segment, and the acenocoumarol group 42%—this difference was not significant.

There were more bleeding complications in the anticoagulant group than in the ticlopidine group. In the latter group, side effects were rare—only three patients discontinued treatment because of gastrointestinal disorders. No particular hematological changes were observed during the follow-up.

Finally, Limet et al.[32] carried out an investigation to evaluate how long ticlopidine treatment could ensure graft patency. They undertook a double-blind, placebo-controlled study, which included 175 patients who had undergone aortocoronary bypass. Each patient was given ticlopidine (250 mg bid) or placebo 48 hours after operation and was followed up for 1 year. Graft patency, which was the primary endpoint of the study, was assessed at 10, 180, and 360 days after operation. Secondary endpoints were instrumental tests, such as exercise evidence of ischemia or infarction, and the analysis of new vascular and non-vascular events. Graft-by-graft analysis showed a lower number of occluded grafts in patients taking ticlopidine than in those given placebo. This difference was observed at day 10 (7.1% vs. 13.4%, $p < 0.05$), day 180 (15% vs. 24%, $p < 0.02$), and day 360 (15% vs. 26%, $p < 0.01$) (Table 7.2).

Patient-by-patient analysis showed a more frequent bypass closure in patients given a placebo than in those given ticlopidine. At rest and during stress, scintigraphy was performed 6 months after operation but no particular differences were observed between the placebo and ticlopidine groups.

During a 1-year follow-up, intercurrent events due predominantly to cardiovascular accidents were registered. Major intercurrent events, including death, myocardial infarction, stroke, at rest-angina, or pulmonary embolism, were 6.9% in the ticlopidine group and 14% in the placebo group.

Clinical side effects were equally distributed between the two groups and included gastrointestinal disturbances, hepatitis, and skin reactions. Four patients in the ticlopidine group and three patients in the placebo group experienced severe neutropenia, causing treatment to be discontinued. The neutrophil count of two patients taking ticlopidine and of one taking placebo dropped below 1,000 per mm^3 but returned quickly to baseline value after interruption of treatment.

Conclusions

When these studies are considered together, they indicate that ticlopidine treatment initiated 24–48 hours after operation significantly reduces early and late closure of vein graft bypass. In most cases treatment was well tolerated, the most frequent side effect being slight gastrointestinal disturbances. Hematological adverse events such as neutropenia were also reported, suggesting that appropriate monitoring should be carried out, in particular during the first months of therapy.

Angioplasty

Physiopathology

In the last decade percutaneous transluminal coronary angioplasty (PTCA) showed an increasing success rate, probably due to an improvement in both operator experience and technical approach. However, two major problems still remain, i.e., early occlusion due to a thrombotic process occurring at the site of angioplasty, and late occlusion caused by a process of restenosis.[28] Early occlusion is a consequence of the deep arterial injury resulting from a fracture of atherosclerotic plaque. This exposes subintimal structures, such as collagen, von Willebrand factor, smooth muscle cells, or release-tissue thromboplastin, which activates coagulation pathways and platelets.[28] Platelet deposition in the angioplastic area is caused by arterial deep injury. Subendothelial injury produces laminar platelet deposition but does not lead to thrombus formation, whereas deep injury produces major platelet deposition and thrombus formation.[28] The latter condition is typical of angioplastic procedures and induces an acute vascular occlusion in about 2–12% of patients. Due to the complex mechanism (coagulation and platelet activation) leading to thrombus formation, immediate use of an anticoagulant, such as heparin, is a routine procedure that tends to limit acute occlusion. This therapeutic approach is based on the assumption that heparin given intravenously inhibits thrombin activation and ultimately limits platelet deposition. In an experimental approach carried out on pigs, Heras et al.[33] showed that platelet deposition is inversely related to heparin dosage, i.e., the higher the dosage of heparin the lower the platelet deposition.

Early limitation of platelet deposition could have clinical relevance since platelets also seem to play a pivotal role in the late occlusion occurring at 2 and 3 months after angioplasty. This phenomenon is evident in about 30% of patients.[34] The anatomic lesion characteristic of restenosis is intimal hyperplasia,

TABLE 7.3. Ticlopidine on the prevention of restenosis after angioplasty.

	Study design	Follow-up	Treatment	Restenosis
White et al.[1]	Randomized	6 months	ASA + DIP	33%
	Double blind		Ticlopidine	39%
			Placebo	25%
Bertrand et al.[1]	Randomized	6 months	Placebo	40.7%
	Double blind		Ticlopidine	49.6%

[1] Both studies documented a significant reduction of acute closure in patients given antiplatelet drugs.
DIP = Dipyridamole.

which is entirely due to proliferation of smooth muscle cells. This reaction is a major factor conditioning the anatomic evolution of the arterial wall: intimal thickening or atherosclerotic plaque leading to dynamically significant lesions representing an extreme aspect of a unique pathogenic mechanism.[34]

As platelets adhere to arterial wall a few minutes after angioplasty, it is conceivable that they play some role in the mechanism leading to intima hyperplasia. Platelets adhering to the subendothelium surface lose 97% of their α-granules within 30 minutes.[34] As most of the constituents of α-granules can be detected throughout the intima and media, it is likely that PGDF, a substance contained in the α-granules with potent mitogenic activity, may also be present in the subendothelium thereby stimulating smooth muscle cell proliferation.[34] Platelets, therefore, might play a crucial role in the arterial changes occurring early and late after angioplasty. The limitation of *in situ* platelet activation, and finally of early or late vascular occlusion, represents the rationale for use of antiplatelet agents after angioplasty.

Clinical Trials with Ticlopidine

The effects of ticlopidine treatment on early and late vascular complications occurring after angioplasty have been assessed in two clinical trials (Table 7.3).

White et al.[35] followed up 333 patients who underwent coronary angioplasty in a double-blind, placebo-controlled study. Patients were given either aspirin (325 mg bid) plus dipyridamole (75 mg tid), ticlopidine (250 mg bid) or placebo 4–5 days before angioplasty. Endpoints of the study were early occlusion and restenosis, the latter being investigated by coronary angiography 6 months after operation. Immediate complications, such as abrupt occlusion, thrombosis, and major dissection, occurred more frequently in the placebo group (14%) than in groups given aspirin plus dipyridamole (5%, $p < 0.005$) or ticlopidine (2%, $p < 0.005$). On the other hand, assessment of coronary restenosis 6 months after angioplasty did not show any effects of the two active regimens. The rate of restenosis was 25% in the placebo group, 33% in the group given aspirin plus dipyridamole and 39% in the group given ticlopidine. Moreover, the two active regimens did not influence late clinical events, such as nonfatal myocardial infarction, or cardiac death occurring after angioplasty. No side effects were reported during the study.

Bertrand et al.[36] supported this finding in a subsequent double-blind clinical trial in which ticlopidine (250 mg bid) or a placebo were administered to 266 patients who had undergone angioplasty. Acute closure and restenosis assessed by coronary angiography 6 months after angioplasty were the major end-points of the study. Acute closure was 16.2% in the placebo group and 5.1% in the ticlopidine group (p < 0.01). However, the antiplatelet treatment did not influence restenosis, which was 40.7% in the placebo group and 49.6% in the ticlopidine group. There was no report of side effects during the study.

Conclusions

Experimental and clinical studies indicate that platelets play a pivotal role in the acute vascular closure that occurs immediately after angioplasty. Anti-platelet treatment with aspirin plus dipyridamole or with ticlopidine clearly demonstrated the beneficial effect of this pharmacological approach, which reduces acute vascular complications. On the other hand, late complications, such as restenosis, do not seem to be affected by antiplatelet treatment, which suggests that more complex mechanisms involving other cellular structures, i.e., endothelium, smooth muscle cell and macrophages, are probably impli-cated in this phenomenon.

References

1. Antiplatelet Trialists' Collaboration. Secondary prevention of vascular disease by prolonged antiplatelet treatment. *Br Med J* 1988;**296**:320–331.
2. Maseri A. Pathogenic classification of unstable angina as a guideline to individual patient management and prognosis. *Am J Med* 1986;**80**:48–55.
3. Falk E. Unstable angina with fatal outcome: dynamic coronary thrombosis leading to infarction and/or sudden death. *Circulation* 1985;**71**:699–708.
4. Duncan B, Fulton M, Morrison SL, Lutz W, Donald KW, Kerr F, Kirby BJ, Julian DG, Oliver FM. Prognosis of new and worsening angina pectoris. *Br Med J* 1976;**1**:981–985.
5. Braunwald E. Unstable angina: a classification. *Circulation* 1989;**80**:410–414.
6. Neill WA, Ritzmann LW, Selden R. The pathophysiologic basis of acute coronary insufficiency: observations favouring the hypothesis of intermittent reversible coronary obstruction. *Am Heart J* 1977;**94**:439–445.
7. Moise A, Theroux P, Taeymans Y, Descoings B, Lesperance Y, Waters DD, Pelletier GB, Bourasse MG. Unstable angina and progression of coronary atherosclerosis. *N Engl J Med* 1983;**309**:685–689.
8. Ambrose JA, Winters SL, Arora RR, Eng A, Ricco A, Gorlin R, Fuster V. Angio-graphic evaluation of coronary artery morphology in unstable angina. *JACC* 1986; **7**:472–478.

9. Fuster V, Badimon L, Cohen M, Ambrose JA, Badimon JJ, Chesebro J. Insights into the pathogenesis of acute ischemic syndromes. *Circulation* 1988;**77**:1213–1220.
10. Falk E. Thrombosis in unstable angina: pathologic aspects. In Metha JL, Conti CR (eds) *Thrombosis and Platelets in Myocardial Ischemia,* FA Davis Company, Philadelphia, 1987, pp 137–149.
11. Sherman CT, Litvack F, Grundfest W, Lee M, Hickey A, Chaux A, Kass R, Blanche C, Matloff J, Morgenstern L, Ganz W, Swan HJC, Forrester J. Coronary angioscopy in patients with unstable angina pectoris. *N Engl J Med* 1986;**315**:913–919.
12. Davies MJ, Thomas AC, Knapman PA, Hangertuer JR. Intramyocardial platelet aggregation in patients with unstable angina suffering sudden ischemic cardiac death. *Circulation* 1986;**73**:418–427.
13. Fitzgerald DJ, Roy L, Catella F, Fitzgerald G. Platelet activation in unstable coronary disease. *N Engl J Med* 1986;**315**:983–989.
14. Vejar M, Fragasso G, Hackett D, et al. Dissociation of platelet activation and spontaneous myocardial ischemia in unstable angina. *Thromb Haemost* 1990;**63**:163–168.
15. Lewis HD, Davis JW, Archibald DG, et al. Protective effects of aspirin against acute myocardial infarction and death in men with unstable angina. *N Engl J Med* 1983;**309**:396–403.
16. Cairns JA, Gent M, Singer J, et al. Aspirin, sulphinpyrazone, or both in unstable angina. *N Engl J Med* 1985;**313**:1396–1475.
17. Harker LA, Fuster V. Pharmacology of platelet inhibitors. *JACC* 1986;**8**:21b–32b.
18. Maffrand JP, Bernat A, Delebassée D, Defreyn G, Cazenave JP, Gordon JL. ADP plays a key role in thrombogenesis in rats. *Thromb Haemost* 1988;**59**:225–230.
19. di Minno G, Cerbone AM, Mattioli PL, Turco S, Iovine C, Mancini M. Functionally thromboasthenic state in normal platelets following the administration of ticlopidine. *J Clin Invest* 1985;**75**:328–338.
20. Panak EA, Maffrand JP, Picard-Fraire C, Vallée E, Blanchard JF, Roncucci R. Ticlopidine: a promise for the prevention and treatment of thrombosis and its complications. *Haemostasis* 1983;**13**(suppl 1):1–54.
21. Theroux P, Ouimet H, McCans J, et al. Aspirin, heparin, or both to treat acute unstable angina. *N Engl J Med* 1988;**319**:1105–1112.
22. RISC Group. Risk of myocardial infarction and death during treatment with low dose aspirin and intravenous heparin in men with unstable coronary artery disease. *Lancet* 1990;**336**:827–830.
23. Balsano F, Rizzon P, Violi F, et al. Study of ticlopidine in unstable angina. *Circulation* 1990;**82**:17–26.
24. Chesebro JH, Fuster V. Role of platelet and platelet inhibitors in aortocoronary artery vein-graft occlusion. *Circulation* 1986;**73**:227–232.
25. Campeen L, Lesperance Y, Grondin CM, Bourasse MG. Angiographic evaluation of post-operative changes in saphenous vein aorto-coronary by-pass graft and coronary arteries. *Prog Cardiol* 1977;**6**:185–211.
26. Josa M, Lia JT, Bianco RL, Kaye M. Reduction of thrombosis in canine coronary bypass vein grafts with dipyridamole and aspirin. *Am J Cardiol* 1981;**47**:1248–54.
27. Unni KK, Kottke BA, Titus JL, et al. Pathologic changes in aortocoronary saphenous vein grafts. *Am J Cardiol* 1974;**34**:526–532.
28. Chesebro JH, Lem JY, Fuster V. The pathogenesis and prevention of aortocoronary vein bypass occlusion and restenosis after arterial angioplasty: role of vascular injury and platelet thrombus deposition. *JACC* 1986;**8**:57b–66b.

29. Walter P, Geronlanos S, Rothlin M, et al. Dierasterelek tronenoposchen Oberflichen-veran-derungen der Gefassunflache gewobener Dacrongefassprothesen uach Varabreichung von Ticlopidine. *Folia Angiol* 1987;**29**:20–32.
30. Chevigné M, David JL, Rigo P, Limet R.Effect of ticlopidine on saphenous vein bypass patency rates: a double-blind study. *Ann Thorac Surg* 1984;**37**:371–378.
31. Rothlin ME, Pflunger N, Speiser K, et al. Platelet inhibitors versus anticoagulants for prevention of aortocoronary bypass graft occlusion. *Eur Heart J* 1985;**6**:168–175.
32. Limet R, David JL, Megotteaux P, Larock MP, Rigo P. Prevention of aorto-coronary bypass graft occlusion. Beneficial effect of ticlopidine on early and late patency rates of venous coronary bypass grafts: a double-blind study. *Ann Thorac Surg* 1987;**94**:773–783.
33. Heras M, Chesebro JH, Penny WJ, et al. Importance of adequate heparin dosage in arterial angioplasty in a porcine model. *Circulation* 1988;**78**:654–660.
34. Lin MW, Ronbin GS, Spencer BK. Restenosis after coronary angioplasty. Potential biologic determinants and role of intimal hyperplasia. *Circulation* 1989;**79**:1357–1387.
35. White CW, Chaitman B, Lasser TA, et al. Antiplatelet agents are effective in reducing the immediate complications of PTCA: results from Ticlopidine Multicenter Study. *Circulation* 1987;**76**(suppl IV):1591.
36. Bertrand ME, Allain H, Lablanche JM, et al. Results of a randomized trial of ticlopidine versus placebo for prevention of acute closure and restenosis after coronary angioplasty (PTCA). The TACT study. XIIth Congress of the European Society of Cardiology. Abstract supplement P2022, 1990.

8
A Systematic Overview of Randomized Trials of Antiplatelet Agents for the Prevention of Stroke, Myocardial Infarction, and Vascular Death

MICHAEL GENT

The established role of platelets in arterial thrombosis has provided the basic rationale for a number of randomized trials of antiplatelet drugs in patients with disorders thought to be associated with platelet thrombi.[1]

Over the past 25 years there have been over 200 randomized trials in more than 100,000 patients exploring the potential clinical benefits of antiplatelet drugs. Drugs studied include aspirin, dipyridamole (nearly always in combination with aspirin), sulfinpyrazone, suloctidil, and ticlopidine. Clinical disorders within which these drugs have been evaluated include transient ischemic attacks (TIAs) or mild stroke; completed stroke; myocardial infarction; unstable angina; coronary artery bypass surgery; coronary angioplasty; heart valve replacement; and peripheral arterial disease. Several studies have also been performed in patient groups at risk of deep vein thrombosis as well as some small studies in patients on hemodialysis or with subarachnoid hemorrhage. Finally, there have been two important studies in primary prevention. Efficacy outcomes have included selected combinations of stroke, myocardial infarction, and death; graft patency; restenosis; venous thromboembolism; and various symptomatology. This chapter will review the key studies in which efficacy outcomes included major vascular ischemic events of stroke, myocardial infarction, and vascular death and establish the current position regarding efficacy and safety of antiplatelet drugs within this context.

Transient Ischemic Attacks and Mild Strokes

The knowledge that the majority of disabling and fatal strokes are thromboembolic and are sometimes preceded by transient ischemic attacks (TIAs)[2] has led to the publication of 22 randomized trials of platelet-inhibiting drugs in nearly 17,000 patients with TIAs or minor strokes.[3-24] In 12 of these trials (Table 8.1), numbers of patients studied and numbers of outcome events observed were relatively small, and while each of these studies represent useful stages in clinical evaluation of antiplatelet drugs, each was too small to have sufficient statistical power to detect an important clinical benefit. The other

TABLE 8.1. Small studies: TIA/mild stroke.

Study	Year	Study drugs	# Patients
Acheson	1969	Dipyridamole	169
Evans	1972	Sulfinpyrazone	23
Fields	1977	ASA	178
Reuther	1978	ASA	58
Fields	1978	ASA	125
Olsson	1980	ASA	135
Roden	1981	Sulfinpyrazone	59
Herskovits	1981	ASA	66
Candelise	1982	ASA/sulfinpyrazone	124
Sorensen	1983	ASA	203
Vinazzer	1987	ASA	60
Boysen	1988	ASA	301

10 studies (Table 8.2) provide the key data on which the current position regarding absolute and relative efficacy of aspirin, dipyridamole, sulfinpyrazone, and ticlopidine should be based.

The Canadian Cooperative Study Group carried out a randomized, placebo-controlled study to assess relative efficacy of aspirin (325 mg qid) and sulfinpyrazone (200 mg qid), singly and in combination, in the reduction of TIAs, stroke or death.[15] Followed for an average of 26 months were 585 patients (70% males) with one or more cerebral or retinal ischemic attacks within 3 months before entry. Aspirin reduced risk of TIA, stroke, or death by 19% (p < 0.05). If only stroke or death were considered, aspirin reduced risk by 31% (p < 0.05). There was no statistically significant reduction in these events attributable to sulfinpyrazone. A striking difference was found between male and female patients in their therapeutic response to aspirin—there was a risk reduction of 48% in stroke or death among men but no observed benefit among women (p = 0.003).

Guiraud-Chaumeil et al. randomly allocated 440 patients presenting with TIAs to one of three treatment groups, all of whom received dihydroergocornine (4.5 g daily); one group received nothing else, one group also received aspirin (300 mg tid), and the third group received aspirin (300 mg tid) plus dipyridamole (50 mg tid).[16] The results of this unblinded trial showed no statistically significant differences among the three treatment groups in incidence of the composite outcome of TIA, stroke, or death over a 3-year follow-up period. The observed rates were 25%, 13%, and 18% in the control, aspirin, and aspirin plus dipyridamole groups, respectively. However, the observed risk reduction with active treatment was nearly 40%.

Bousser et al. carried out a randomized double-blind, placebo-controlled trial in 604 patients with TIA or minor stroke in the preceding year to assess treatment effects for 3 years with aspirin (325 mg tid) or the combination of aspirin (325 mg tid) plus dipyridamole (75 mg tid).[17] The number of fatal or nonfatal cerebral infarctions was 31 in the placebo group, 17 in the aspirin group, and 18 in the

TABLE 8.2. Major studies: TIA/mild stroke.

Study	Year	Study drugs	# Patients
Barnett	1978	ASA/sulfinpyrazone	585
Guiraud-Cha umeil	1982	ASA/dipridamole	440
Bousser	1983	ASA/dipyridamole	604
Tohgi	1984	ASA/ticlopidine	340
Fields	1985	ASA/dipyridamole	890
ESPS	1987	ASA/dipyridamole	2500
UKTIA	1988	ASA	2435
TASS	1989	ASA/ticlopidine	3069
Dutch	1991	ASA	3131
SALT	1991	ASA	1360

combination aspirin–dipyridamole group, corresponding to cumulative rates of 18% in the placebo group, and 10.5% in each of the active treatment groups. The observed risk reduction with active treatment was 41% ($p = 0.02$). Myocardial infarction was less in the active treatment groups than in placebo (3% vs. 9%; $p < 0.05$). Side effects, particularly symptoms of peptic ulcer and hemorrhagic events sufficient to cause permanent discontinuation of study drug, were significantly more frequent in the two groups containing aspirin (9% vs. 3%; $p < 0.01$).

In the UK-TIA study, 2435 patients with a recent TIA or minor ischemic stroke were randomly allocated in a double-blind manner to receive aspirin (600 mg bid), aspirin (300 mg daily) or placebo.[18] The mean follow-up was 4 years. Risk of stroke, myocardial infarction, or death was 18% lower in each of the two aspirin groups relative to the placebo group ($2p = 0.01$). The lower dose of aspirin was significantly less gastrotoxic than the higher dose. Incidence of bleeding was 2.5%, 4.1%, and 7.0%, respectively, in the placebo group, lower-dose aspirin group, and higher-dose aspirin group.

SALT was a randomized, double-blind trial to assess efficacy of 75 mg aspirin daily in the prevention of stroke or death in patients with recent (1–4 months) TIAs or minor stroke.[19] Based on a median follow-up of 32 months on 1360 patients, the aspirin group showed a reduction of 18% in risk of stroke or death ($p = 0.02$), which was similar for males and females. Risk reduction in the combined outcome of the first event of stroke, myocardial infarction, or vascular death was 17% ($p = 0.03$). Gastrointestinal side effects were only slightly more common in the aspirin-treated patients, but there was a significant excess of severe bleeding episodes (3.0% vs. 1.3%).

The Dutch TIA trial compared the effects of two doses of aspirin (30 mg vs. 283 mg daily) on the incidence of stroke, myocardial infarction, or vascular death in 3131 patients with recent TIA or minor ischemic stroke.[20] The mean follow-up was 31 months. Incidence of primary efficacy outcome was 14.7% and 15.2% in the lower and higher dose groups, respectively. Correspondingly, there was also little difference in proportions of patients reporting gastrointestinal symptoms

(10.5% vs. 11.4%). There were slightly fewer major bleeding complications in the 30 mg group (40 vs. 53).

The European Stroke Prevention Study (ESPS) Group carried out a double-blind trial in which 2500 patients with a clinical diagnosis of a recent TIA, reversible ischemic neurological deficit (RIND), or stroke were randomized to receive either aspirin (325 mg tid) plus dipyridamole (75 mg tid) or identical placebos. Follow-up was 24 months.[21] In an intention-to-treat analysis, there was a 33% risk reduction in stroke or death from any cause with active treatment (p < 0.001). Side effects were the main reason for permanent discontinuation of study drug in 13.1% of patients on aspirin plus dipyridamole and 6.7% on placebo (p < 0.001). Reports of gastrointestinal complaints were much more frequent on the active regimen (711 vs. 445) as were reports of bleeding (91 vs. 48).

The American-Canadian Cooperative Study Group carried out a randomized, double-blind trial in 890 patients with a recent TIA to assess relative efficacy of aspirin (325 mg qid) and aspirin (325 mg qid) plus dipyridamole (75 mg qid) in reducing risk of cerebral or retinal infarction, or death.[22] Median follow-up was about 3 years. The number of observed efficacy outcomes was 84 in the aspirin group and 85 in the aspirin plus dipyridamole group, and the corresponding 3-year rates were 21.6% and 21.8%, respectively. Peptic ulcer developed in 24 patients on aspirin alone and 20 on the combination regimen; corresponding numbers for hemorrhagic side effects were 36 and 32, respectively.

Tohgi compared 12 months of treatment with aspirin (500 mg daily) or ticlopidine (200 mg daily) in a randomized, double-blind trial in 340 patients with a TIA in the previous 3 months.[23] Incidence of TIAs, RIND, cerebral infarction, or myocardial infarction was 29.6% in the aspirin group compared with 19.4% in the ticlopidine group (p > 0.05), with the vast majority of events being TIAs. Corresponding rates excluding TIAs were 8.9% and 4.8%

The Ticlopidine Aspirin Stroke Study (TASS) was a randomized, double-blind trial to evaluate relative risk reduction in stroke or death from any cause conferred by ticlopidine (250 bid) compared to aspirin (650 mg bid) in patients who had experienced TIA, RIND, or minor stroke within the previous 3 months.[24] Fifty-six centers in North America recruited 3069 patients who were followed up to 5.8 years (mean 3.3 years). A significant benefit of ticlopidine over aspirin was observed in the intention-to-treat analysis: a 12% relative risk reduction in the incidence of stroke or death from any cause (2p = 0.048) and a 20% relative risk reduction in the incidence of fatal or nonfatal stroke (2p = 0.024) were recorded over the first 3 years. The relative benefit of ticlopidine was seen in both males and females. Adverse effects of aspirin included gastritis, peptic ulceration and gastrointestinal bleeding. Diarrhea, skin rashes and a severe but reversible neutropenia (less than 1%), were noted with ticlopidine treatment.

In considering all the above findings, it would be reasonable to conclude that aspirin is efficacious, since a statistically significant and clinically important benefit was found independently in three studies.[15,18,19] Furthermore, the findings from two other studies were consistent with this conclusion.[16,17] It would be

TABLE 8.3. Studies: moderate/severe stroke.

Study	Year	Study drugs	# Patients
Blakely	1975	Sulfinpyrazone	99
Blakely	1979	Sulfinpyrazone	290
Gent	1985	Suloctidil	447
Swedish	1987	ASA	505
CATS	1989	Ticlopidine	1072
ESPS	1990	ASA/dipyridamole	1502

difficult, however, to conclude from these five studies, together with the Dutch study,[20] what the optimal dose of aspirin should be. ESPS provided strong evidence that the combination of aspirin plus dipyridamole is efficacious but does not address the question of whether or not it is more efficacious than aspirin alone. Within each of the three studies in which these two regimens were compared directly,[16,17,22] the observed rates at which efficacy outcomes occurred in the two treatment groups were almost identical. Hence, there is no evidence that addition of dipyridamole to aspirin provides any benefit over that of aspirin alone. There was no demonstrable benefit of sulfinpyrazone in the one study in which it was evaluated.[15] The TASS findings[24] suggest that ticlopidine may be better than aspirin and should certainly be considered as the only drug along with aspirin that has been shown to be of benefit in patients with recent TIAs or mild stroke.

Moderate/Severe Strokes

There have been five randomized trials evaluating antiplatelet drugs restricted to patients with recent moderate/severe ischemic stroke (Table 8.3),[25–29] and one study with a large subgroup of such patients on whom outcomes were reported separately from those patients in the same study with TIA or mild stroke.[30]

Blakely and Gent carried out a randomized, double-blind study of sulfinpyrazone (200 mg tid) in 291 institutionalized elderly patients to evaluate the effect of mortality compared with placebo.[25] In a subgroup of 99 patients with a previously documented stroke, mortality from all causes was significantly reduced in the sulfinpyrazone group, the reduction being most marked in the frequency of death from vascular causes. In a subsequent randomized trial in 290 patients with thrombotic stroke in which the observed risk reduction in mortality was 13% (p > 0.1),[26] Blakely was unable to confirm a real benefit of sulfinpyrazone.

Gent et al. reported a randomized double-blind, placebo-controlled trial to assess the benefit of suloctidil (200 mg bid) in 438 patients with a thromboembolic stroke within the previous 4 months.[27] There was an observed reduction of 24% in risk of stroke, myocardial infarction, or vascular death in the suloctidil group relative to the placebo group, which was not statistically significant. The study was stopped sooner than planned because suloctidil was found to be hepatotoxic.

The Swedish Cooperative Study Group randomized 505 patients who had had a minor or major stroke in the previous 3 weeks to either aspirin (1500 mg daily) or matching placebo and followed them for 2 years.[28] Incidence of outcome events in the active and placebo groups, respectively, were 23% and 22% for stroke or death from any cause and 12% and 13% for stroke alone. Permanent withdrawal from study drug because of side effects occurred in 32 patients in the aspirin group compared to 21 patients in the placebo group (p < 0.05).

The Canadian American Ticlopidine Study (CATS) was a randomized double-blind, placebo-controlled trial to assess ticlopidine's benefit (250 mg bid) in reducing risk of stroke, myocardial infarction, or vascular death in patients who had suffered a recent (1 week to 4 months) thromboembolic stroke.[29] For this trial, 1072 patients were enrolled in 25 clinical centers and were treated and followed for up to 3 years (mean 24 months). In the primary analysis of efficacy, the event rate per year for the above cluster of outcomes was 15.3% in the placebo group and 10.8% in the ticlopidine group, representing a relative risk reduction with ticlopidine of 30% (p = 0.006). A similar, statistically significant benefit was observed in both men and women. Adverse experiences associated with ticlopidine included diarrhea, skin rash and neutropenia (severe in less than 1% of cases) that were always reversible.

The ESPS Group reported a more detailed analysis of their study and, in particular, provided an analysis relating to 1502 patients whose deficit persisted for more than 7 days and could reasonably be classified as moderate/severe strokes.[30] Incidence of stroke or death was 26.6% in the placebo group and 18.1% in the aspirin plus dipyridamole group, representing a relative risk reduction of 32.3% (p < 0.001).

Based simply on the above six studies alone, one could reasonably come to the conclusion that neither sulfinpyrazone nor aspirin have been shown to be of benefit in patients with moderate/severe stroke and that there is a persuasive evidence that both aspirin plus dipyridamole and ticlopidine are efficacious.

Myocardial Infarction

Elwood et al. reported a randomized, placebo-controlled study of aspirin (300 mg daily) in 1239 men with a recent myocardial infarction.[31] There was an observed risk reduction of 25% in death from any cause after 1 year that was not statistically significant. However, for those randomized within 6 weeks of their qualifying infarction, there was a statistically significant observed reduction in mortality from 13.2% in the placebo group to 7.8% in the aspirin group. There was little difference reported in the incidence of side effects.

The Coronary Drug Project Research Group reported a randomized, placebo-controlled trial in 1529 men who had had a myocardial infarction about 7 years previously and who had been participants in two other secondary prevention studies that had been terminated.[32] Over an average of 20 months of follow-up, those randomized to aspirin (325 mg tid) had a mortality of 5.8% compared to 8.3% in the placebo group, an observed risk reduction of 30%, which is clinically impressive but not statistically significant.

Elwood and Sweetman randomized 1682 patients with a confirmed myocardial infarction, mostly within a week, to receive either aspirin (300 mg tid) or matching placebo.[33] Patients were treated and followed for 1 year. Overall mortality was 12.3% in patients given aspirin and 14.8% in the placebo group, a relative risk reduction of 17%. The corresponding reduction for mortality due to ischemic heart disease was 22%—neither of these risk reductions was statistically significant. For the combined outcome of death or nonfatal myocardial infarction, risk reduction was 28% (p < 0.05).

Breddin et al. randomly allocated 946 patients within 6 weeks of their myocardial infarction to aspirin (500 mg tid), a placebo (making the assessment of aspirin's benefit double-blind) or to phenprocoumon and followed them for up to 2 years.[34] There was little difference in overall mortality, but the coronary death rate (sudden death or fatal myocardial infarction), while not significantly different, was only 4.1% in the aspirin-treated patients compared to 7.1% in the placebo group, a relative risk reduction of 42%.

The Aspirin Myocardial Infarction Study Research Group carried out a randomized, placebo-controlled trial in 4524 patients with a documented myocardial infarction 2 to 60 months previously who were treated and followed for up to 3 years.[35] Overall mortality in the aspirin (500 mg bid) group was 10.8% compared to 9.7% in the placebo group. Corresponding rates for coronary incidence (coronary death or nonfatal myocardial infarction) were 14.1% and 14.8%, respectively. Symptoms suggestive of peptic ulcer, gastritis, or erosion of gastric mucosa occurred in 23.7% of the aspirin group and 14.9% of the placebo group.

The Persantine-Aspirin Reinfarction Study Research Group recruited 2206 patients with a documented myocardial infarction within the past 2 to 60 months and randomly allocated them to aspirin (324 mg tid), aspirin (324 mg tid) plus dipyridamole (75 mg tid) or placebo, with twice as many patients in each of the active-treatment groups, and followed them for 41 months on average.[36] Overall mortality, coronary heart disease mortality, and coronary incidence were quite similar in the two active-treatment groups and consistently less than in the placebo group. For none of these outcome events was the observed difference statistically significant. Symptoms suggestive of peptic ulcer, gastritis, or erosion of gastric mucosa were reported in 19.4% of the active-treatment groups and 13.2% of the placebo group.

Thus, by this time there had been six major randomized trials evaluating aspirin's efficacy and safety in more than 10,000 myocardial infarction patients, over 1000 of whom died during the study, and yet without one of them demonstrating a statistically significant benefit. Five studies had shown a trend in favor

TABLE 8.4. Early aspirin studies postmyocardial infarction.

Study	Year	# Patients
Elwood	1974	1239
CDP	1975	1529
German-Austrian	1977	626
Elwood	1979	1759
AMIS	1980	4524
PARIS	1980	1216
Total		10,893

Cardiovascular death: 16% risk reduction (p < 0.01).
Reinfarction (fatal or nonfatal): 21% risk reduction (p < 0.0001).

of aspirin therapy; in contrast, the largest study showed no evidence of benefit. However, a subsequent analysis by Peto, in which the results of these six studies were combined, indicated that there was an overall significant benefit of aspirin (Table 8.4).[37] He reported that for cardiovascular death, the pooled estimate of risk reduction with aspirin was 16% (p < 0.01), and for the outcome of myocardial infarction the risk reduction with aspirin was 21% (p < 0.001).

This benefit of aspirin was confirmed by ISIS-2 (the Second International Study of Infarct Survival), in which 17,187 patients with suspected acute myocardial infarction were randomized to receive enteric-coated aspirin (162 mg daily) for 1 month, a single dose of streptokinase, both, or neither.[38] The 5-week vascular mortality was 9.4% in patients treated with aspirin and 11.8% in patients not treated with aspirin, a relative risk reduction of 23% (2p < 0.00001). Differences in vascular and all-cause mortality produced by aspirin remained highly significant (2p < 0.001) after a median follow-up of 15 months. Aspirin significantly reduced both nonfatal reinfarction and nonfatal stroke, each by nearly 50%. Aspirin was not associated with any significant increase in cerebral hemorrhage or in bleeds requiring transfusion.

In the Persantine-Aspirin Reinfarction Study Part II, 3128 patients with a myocardial infarction sustained 4 weeks to 4 months previously, were randomized to receive either aspirin (325 mg tid) plus dipyridamole (75 mg tid) or matching placebo.[39] The average length of follow-up was 23 months. There was a relative risk reduction of 30% in coronary incidence (nonfatal myocardial infarction or cardiac death) at 1 year with active treatment and 24% over the course of the study; both of these were statistically significant (p < 0.01). Corresponding reductions for coronary mortality were 20% and 6%, neither of which was statistically significant. Gastrointestinal symptoms and bleeding were twice as common in the active treatment group.

The Anturane Reinfarction Trial Research Group reported the initial findings of a trial in which patients were randomly allocated to sulfinpyrazone (200 mg qid) or placebo 25 to 35 days after a myocardial infarction and showed a statistically significant reduction in cardiac mortality from 9.5% per year to

4.9%.[40] Patient recruitment stopped at that time, but follow-up was continued until all 1558 eligible patients had completed at least 1 year of follow-up. Based on an average follow-up of 16 months, a second report showed an overall reduction of 32% in cardiac mortality (p = 0.06), which was due almost entirely to a 75% reduction in sudden death over the first 6 months of treatment (p = 0.003), after which time there seemed to be no further benefit of treatment.[41] Apart from a small excess of gastrointestinal symptoms (28% vs. 23%), there was virtually no difference between the two groups in newly observed signs or symptoms. Following a critique by the FDA,[42] the study group reported a further analysis with findings similar to the earlier ones,[43] but controversy remained.[44]

The Anturane Reinfarction Italian Study Group randomly allocated 727 patients within 15 to 25 days following an acute myocardial infarction to either sulfinpyrazone (400 mg bid) or matching placebo and followed them for up to 4 years and for 19 months on average.[45] There were 15 reinfarctions, fatal or nonfatal, in the sulfinpyrazone group compared with 34 in the placebo group; this represents a relative risk reduction of 56% (p < 0.005). Vascular death was similar in the two groups. Sulfinpyrazone was well tolerated with no excess side effects over placebo.

On the basis of these studies there is strong evidence that aspirin is of benefit in patients with a recent myocardial infarction. There is only limited data on whether there is any real gain in adding dipyridamole to aspirin, and sulfinpyrazone is also beneficial.

Unstable Angina

Lewis and colleagues carried out a randomized double-blind, placebo-controlled trial of aspirin (324 mg in buffered solution once daily) for 12 weeks in 1266 men with unstable angina.[46] Frequency of death or acute myocardial infarction after 3 months was 10.1% in the placebo group and 5.0% in the aspirin group, a relative risk reduction of 51% (p = 0.0005). There was a similar risk reduction in all-cause mortality. There was no difference in gastrointestinal symptoms or bleeding between the two treatment groups. Follow-up at 1 year was achieved in 86% of the patients surviving 12 weeks. Among these patients mean mortality rate in the aspirin group (5.5%) was less than that in the placebo group (9.6%), with a risk reduction of 43% (p = 0.008).

Cairns and colleagues carried out a randomized double-blind, placebo-controlled trial comparing effects of aspirin (325 mg qid) and sulfinpyrazone (200 mg qid), either singly or in combination, with respect to the incidence of subsequent myocardial infarction or cardiac death.[47] Patients were followed for up to 2 years, with a mean of 19 months, and primary efficacy analysis was based on eligible patients who had not been off medication for more than 28 consecutive days preceding an outcome. There was no observed benefit of sulfinpyrazone. However, among patients receiving aspirin, there was an observed

55% risk reduction in myocardial infarction or cardiac death compared with patients not receiving aspirin (p = 0.004). The corresponding risk reduction for death from any cause was 70% (p = 0.005). On an intention-to-treat basis there was a 43% risk reduction for all-cause mortality (p = 0.036). Observed benefits were similar for males and females.

Theroux et al. randomized 479 patients hospitalized with unstable angina to receive aspirin (325 mg bid) or intravenous heparin, both or neither for about 6 days.[48] Incidence of the primary outcome cluster of refractory angina, myocardial infarction, or death was 14.0% in those receiving aspirin and 17.8% in those who did not, a relative risk reduction of 21%, which was not statistically significant. A reduction of 61% with aspirin in the risk of myocardial infarction was statistically significant.

The RISC Group reported a randomized, placebo-controlled study of 796 men with unstable coronary artery disease who received either aspirin (75 mg daily) for up to 1 year, intermittent intravenous heparin for 5 days, both, or neither.[49] The risk of myocardial infarction or death in patients who did not receive aspirin was 5.8% after 5 days, 13.4% after 1 month, and 17.1% after 3 months. Treatment with aspirin reduced these event rates by 57–69%. Hematological side effects due to aspirin were rare and minor.

The Studio della Ticlopidine nell'Angina Instabile (STAI) group reported an open study in which 652 patients with unstable angina were randomized to receive conventional care or to ticlopidine (250 mg bid) in addition to conventional care for a study duration of 6 months.[50] Incidence of myocardial infarction in the conventional care group was 10.9% and 4.7% for vascular death. Corresponding rates in the ticlopidine group were 5.1% and 2.5%, representing relative risk reductions of 53% (p = 0.006) and 47% (p = 0.14), respectively. There were few adverse events in the ticlopidine group and no clinically important changes in the white cell count.

On the basis of these studies in patients with unstable angina, there is again strong evidence of aspirin's benefit as well as ticlopidine's.

Atherosclerotic Peripheral Arterial Disease

There have been two randomized trials of aspirin, with and without dipyridamole, suggesting delay in progression of peripheral occlusive arterial disease, but both studies were too small to assess any benefit in reducing risk of subsequent major vascular ischemic events.[51,52]

Meta-analysis of a number of short-term studies evaluating ticlopidine in patients with atherosclerotic peripheral arterial disease showed a highly significant reduction in fatal or nonfatal vascular events from 9% to 3% (p = 0.006).[53]

The Swedish Ticlopidine Multicentre Study (STIMS) was a placebo-controlled trial to assess efficacy and safety of ticlopidine (250 mg bid) in reducing the incidence of TIA, stroke, and myocardial infarction in patients with intermittent claudication.[54] A total of 687 patients were treated and followed for a median duration of 5.6 years. Allocation to treatment group was by a minimization procedure. There was an 11.4% risk reduction in the primary outcome cluster, a 29% risk reduction in all-cause mortality (p = 0.015), and a 26% risk reduction in vascular death (p < 0.01).

At this time, therefore, only ticlopidine has been shown to be of benefit in reducing vascular ischemic events in patients with peripheral arterial disease.

Primary Prevention

There have been two major randomized trials of the primary prevention of occlusive vascular disease with aspirin. The U.S. Physicians' Health Study was a randomized, placebo-controlled trial of aspirin (325 mg every other day) with 22,071 male physicians, initially 40–84 years of age, who were followed for 60 months on average.[55,56] Aspirin resulted in a 44% relative reduction in the risk of myocardial infarction (p < 0.00001), no reduction in cardiovascular death, and there was a small but not statistically significant increase in stroke. The British Doctors' Trial randomized 5139 male physicians, initially 50–78 years of age, to receive aspirin (500 mg daily) or nothing and were followed for up to 6 years.[57] There was no significant difference for the outcome cluster of stroke, myocardial infarction, or vascular death, nor was there any difference for individual outcomes. A pooled analysis of these two studies showed no significant difference in cardiovascular mortality but a 33% risk reduction in nonfatal myocardial infarction (p < 0.0002).[58]

Overview Analyses

The above reviews are reasonably conventional and provide necessary information for neurologists who have the primary responsibility for prevention and management of strokes and who need to see key data from studies in patients with cerebrovascular disease. The same reasoning applies to a cardiologist who see patients with heart disease. However, it is not enough since the overall conclusions are essentially qualitative rather than quantitative. What is also required is an objective method of combining efficacy data across studies to provide an overall single efficacy estimate. The basic principle in pooling data from several independent randomized trials is to develop a clinically appropriate estimate of efficacy for each trial (e.g., some measure of relative risk reduction) and then to combine these across studies in an unbiased fashion. The method is quite robust with respect to tolerating reasonable heterogeneity among the protocols of the various studies. This strategy requires a common choice of outcome events and specific criteria for selecting studies to be included.

TABLE 8.5. Meta-analysis of three major studies with inactive-control: outcome stroke/MI/vascular death. RR = Risk Reduction

	Placebo	Ticlopidine	Total
CATS (RR = 0.26)			
Outcome	137	107	244
No outcome	404	424	828
Total	541	531	1072
STIMS (RR = 0.26)			
Outcome	103	84	187
No outcome	238	262	500
Total	341	346	687
STAI (RR = 0.51)			
Outcome	47	23	70
No outcome	291	291	582
Total	338	314	652

Pooled analysis: RR = 0.30 (p = 0.0002).

Outcomes chosen for efficacy analyses in the 27 randomized trials of anti-platelet drugs in cerebrovascular disease included such clusters as TIA, stroke, or death; nonfatal or fatal stroke; or, most commonly, stroke or death from any cause. While each of these clusters is reasonable, the current view is most supportive of the outcome cluster of ischemic stroke, myocardial infarction, or vascular death. This cluster has the advantage of adding a major clinical outcome, myocardial infarction, and excluding a probably irrelevant one, nonvascular death. Myocardial infarction is relatively common among patients with ischemic cerebrovascular disease and its risk of occurring is known to be reduced by antiplatelet drugs. On the other hand, nonvascular death is unlikely to be influenced by antiplatelet drugs and its inclusion in the primary cluster of outcomes would simply make it more difficult to demonstrate a true benefit of treatment.

In considering which studies should be included in estimating the absolute and relative efficacy of various antiplatelet drugs in reducing risk of stroke, myocardial infarction, or vascular death, we need to determine which patients are at risk for these major vascular ischemic events. While, traditionally, thrombo-embolic complications of atherosclerosis have been studied in discrete patient groups, defined by focal site of the disease manifestations, there are strong clinical and biological arguments that it is the underlying process that puts patients at risk. Hence, it is reasonable to expect that if antiplatelet drugs can reduce clinical thrombosis, they would be of benefit in preventing vascular ischemic events in a broad spectrum of patients. Such patients would include not only those with ischemic cerebrovascular disease but also those with ischemic cardiac disease and those with atherosclerotic peripheral arterial disease.

As an example, Table 8.5 presents a summary of the number of patients who experienced an outcome of stroke, myocardial infarction, or vascular death, on an intention-to-treat basis, in each of the three major ticlopidine studies without

TABLE 8.6. Meta-analysis of three major studies with inactive-control: outcome vascular death. RR = Risk Reduction

	Placebo	Ticlopidine	Total
CATS (RR = 0.22)			
Outcome	41	32	73
No outcome	500	499	999
Total	541	531	1072
STIMS (RR = 0.43)			
Outcome	58	36	94
No outcome	283	310	593
Total	341	346	687
STAI (RR = 0.44)			
Outcome	15	8	23
No outcome	323	306	629
Total	338	314	652

Pooled analysis: RR = 0.36 (p = 0.0023).

an active control group. Relative risk reductions for CATS, STIMS, and STAI are 26%, 26%, and 57%, respectively, and when these are combined appropriately in a meta-analysis,[59] the overall estimate of ticlopidine's benefit is a relative reduction of 30% in risk of stroke, myocardial infarction, or vascular death (p = 0.0002).

A review of mortality in these three studies would show 170 total deaths in the control group and only 138 in the ticlopidine group. Furthermore, the number of nonvascular deaths is fairly similar in the two groups (56 vs. 62), so that the real difference is in vascular death, as one might expect. Table 8.6 shows the result of a meta-analysis of these studies using vascular death as the outcome; the overall risk reduction in vascular mortality with ticlopidine is 36% (p = 0.0023).

Fortunately, investigators who have been involved in the clinical evaluation of antiplatelet drugs have agreed to form the Antiplatelet Trialists' Collaboration and to share appropriate data from their published and unpublished studies. The first publication from this group included a meta-analysis of 25 randomized trials, including 29,000 patients with histories of cerebral or cardiac disease.[59] The conclusion from this meta-analysis was that the incidence of stroke, myocardial infarction, or vascular death was reduced by about 25% with antiplatelet drugs, and that there was no significant difference between effects of the different types of antiplatelet treatment tested nor between effects in different types of patients.

The most compelling overall assessment of the clinical benefit of antiplatelet drugs will come from the next publication of the Antiplatelet Trialists' Collaboration. At a meeting of this group in Oxford in March 1990, a metaanalysis of nearly 200 randomized trials, including more than 100,000 patients, was presented and showed clearly that antiplatelet drugs are efficacious in reducing the incidence of stroke, myocardial infarction, or vascular death in patients at increased risk of such events, irrespective of their specific clinical manifestations or risk profile. Assessment of efficacy, as measured by relative risk reduction, was remarkably consistent at about 25% across a broad spectrum of clinical disorders and among different subgroups of patients with the same clinical disorders. Hence, on the basis of published studies limited to patients with moderate or severe completed stroke, one could not conclude that aspirin is efficacious in such patients,[60] current evidence overall would suggest that it is. Similarly, aspirin has not been shown directly to be of benefit in reducing risk of subsequent vascular ischemic events in patients with peripheral arterial disease; however, it would be reasonable to assume that it is of benefit.

The next report of the Antiplatelet Trialists' Collaboration will also show that aspirin is clearly of benefit; the combination of aspirin plus dipyridamole is no better than aspirin alone; sulfinpyrazone is unlikely to be better than aspirin; suloctidil is no longer available because of its toxicity; and ticlopidine may be better than aspirin. Thus, there is good evidence that both aspirin and ticlopidine are of benefit in patients with atherosclerotic disease who are at high risk of vascular ischemic events, and they are likely to be more efficacious than the other antiplatelet drugs tested to date.

The majority of clinical studies have used a dose of aspirin of 325 mg daily or more, with a range of 30–1500 mg daily. A Consensus Conference on Antithrombotic Therapy critically reviewed available evidence on aspirin's mechanism of action, on its adverse effects and on its clinical benefit, and concluded that aspirin, in a dose of 325 mg/day, is indicated in patients with acute myocardial infarction or unstable angina.[61] At a recent update meeting of this same international consensus group, the conclusion was that the single overall best estimate of aspirin dose that has consistently been shown to be truly efficacious across a broad spectrum of patients (e.g., TIA, stroke, myocardial infarction, unstable angina, nonvalvular atrial fibrillation) is 325 mg daily. Others have independently advocated the use of 160 mg or 325 mg of aspirin daily in patients with clinical manifestations or coronary disease.[62] These doses are equally effective to higher doses in inhibiting cyclooxygenase-dependent platelet aggregation while having a reduced effect on prostacyclin synthesis in vascular endothelial cells.[63,64]

Many studies with aspirin in patients at risk of vascular ischemic events have used a dose of 1 g/day or more, which is known to produce significant gastrointestinal adverse effects and bleeding. However, there is good evidence that these side effects are dose-related and can be reduced appreciably by using lower doses of 325 mg/day or 160 mg/day.[18,65] What is still debatable is whether or not lower doses of aspirin are significantly safer than 325 mg daily. The only major study with relevant information is the Dutch TIA study, which compared 30 mg with 283 mg of aspirin daily. There was virtually no difference in the proportion of patients reporting gastrointestinal symptoms (10.5% vs. 11.4%), and there were only "...slightly fewer major bleeding complications..." with the lower dose. Therefore, one could not claim to be putting patients at risk by using a dose of 325 mg aspirin daily.

For efficacy, there is no biologic evidence of a dose effect in this range, nor is there strong clinical evidence; however, there is insufficient evidence at this time to be confident that lower doses of aspirin (100 mg daily) are truly as beneficial as doses of 325 mg daily or more. On the other hand, there is good evidence of increased side effects (gastrointestinal and bleeding) with doses higher than 325 mg daily and limited evidence that lower doses are safer. Hence, 325 mg daily is a reasonable dose of aspirin to use in the prevention of vascular ischemic events.

References

1. Didisheim P, Kazmier JF, Fuster V. Platelet inhibition in the management of thrombosis. *Thrombos Diathes Haemorrh* 1974;**32**:21–34.
2. Barnett HJM. The pathophysiology of transient cerebral ischemic attacks. Therapy with platelet antiaggregants. *Med Clin North Am* 1979;**63**:649–679.
3. Acheson J, Danta G, Hutchinson EC. Controlled trial of dipyridamole in cerebral vascular disease. *Br Med J* 1969;1:614–615.
4. Evans G. Effect of drugs that suppress platelet surface interaction on incidence of amaurosis fugax and transient cerebral ischemia. *Surg Forum* 1972;**23**:239–241.
5. Fields WS, Lemak NA, Frankowski RF, Hardy RJ. Controlled trial of aspirin in cerebral ischemia. *Stroke* 1977;**8**:301–316.
6. Reuther R, Dorndorf W. Aspirin in patients with cerebral ischemia and normal angiograms or non surgical lesions. Results of a double blind trial. In Breddin K, Dorndorf W, Loew D, Marx R (eds), *Acetylsalicylic Acid in Cerebral Ischemia and Coronary Heart Disease*. FK Schattauer Verlag, Stuttgart-New York, 1978, pp 97–106.
7. Fields WS, Lemak NA, Frankowski RF, Hardy RJ. Controlled trial of aspirin in cerebral ischemia. Part II: Surgical group. *Stroke* 1978;**9**:309–319.
8. Olsson J-E, Brechter C, Backlund H, et al. Anticoagulant vs. anti-platelet therapy as prophylactic against cerebral infarction in transient ischemic attacks. *Stroke* 1980;**11**:4–9.
9. Roden S, Low-Beer T, Carmalt M, Cockel R, Green I. Transient cerebral ischaemic attacks—management and prognosis. *Postgrad Med J* 1981;**57**:275–278.
10. Herskovits E, Vazquez A, Famulari A, et al. Randomised trial of pentoxifylline versus acetylsalicylic acid plus dipyridamole in preventing transient ischaemic attacks. *Lancet* 1981;1:966–968.
11. Sorensen PS, Pedersen H, Marquardsen J, et al. Acetylsalicylic acid in the prevention of stroke in patients with reversible cerebral ischemic attacks. A Danish cooperative study. *Stroke* 1983;;**14**:15–22.
12. Candelise L, Landi G, Perrone P, Bracchi M, Brambilla G. A randomized trial of aspirin and sulfinpyrazone in patients with TIA. *Stroke* 1982;**13**:175–179.
13. Vinazzer H. Rezidivprophylaxe zerebrovaskulärer Thrombosen. Eine randomisierte Vergleichsstudie mit Azetylsalizylsäure und Natrium-Pentosanpolysulfat. *Fortschr Med* 1987;**105**:79–85.
14. Boysen G, Soelberg-Sorensen P, Juhler M, et al. Danish very-low-dose aspirin after carotid endarterectomy trial. *Stroke* 1988;**19**:1211–1215.
15. The Canadian Cooperative Study Group. A randomized trial of aspirin and sulfinpyrazone in threatened stroke. *N Engl J Med* 1978;**299**:53–59.

16. Guiraud-Chaumeil B, Rascol A, David J, Boneu B, Clanet M, Bierme R. Prévention des récidives des accidents vasculaires cérébraux ischémiques par les anti-agrégants plaquettaires. Résultats d'un essai thérapeutique controlé de 3 ans. *Rev Neurol (Paris)* 1982;**138**:367–385.

17. Bousser MG, Eschwège E, Haguenau M, et al. "AICLA" controlled trial of aspirin and dipyridamole in the secondary prevention of athero-thrombotic cerebral ischemia. *Stroke* 1983;**14**:5–14.

18. UK-TIA Study Group. United Kingdom Transient Ischemic Attack (UK-TIA) aspirin trial; interim results. *Br Med J* 1988;**296**:316–320.

19. The SALT Collaborative Group. Swedish Aspirin Low-dose Trial (SALT) of 75 mg aspirin as secondary prophylaxis after cerebrovascular ischemic events. *Lancet* 1991;**338**:1345–1349.

20. The Dutch TIA Trial Study Group. A comparison of two doses of aspirin (30 mg vs. 283 mg a day) in patients after a transient ischemic attack or minor ischemic stroke. *N Engl J Med* 1991;**325**:1261–1266.

21. ESPS Group. The European Stroke Prevention Study (ESPS); principal endpoints. *Lancet* 1987;**2**:1351–1354.

22. American-Canadian Cooperative Study Group. Persantine aspirin trial in cerebral ischemia. Part II. Endpoint results. *Stroke* 1985;**16**:406–415.

23. Tohgi H. The effect of ticlopidine on TIA compared with aspirin: a double-blind, twelve-month follow-up study. *Agents and Actions Suppl* 1984;**15**:279–282.

24. Hass WK, Easton JD, Adams HP, et al. A randomized trial comparing ticlopidine hydrochloride with aspirin for the prevention of stroke in high-risk patients. *N Engl J Med* 1989;**321**:501–507.

25. Blakely JA, Gent M. Platelets, drugs and longevity in a geriatric population. In Hirsh J, (ed), *Platelets, Drugs and Thrombosis*. S Karger, Basel. 1975, pp 284–291.

26. Blakely JA. A prospective trial of sulfinpyrazone and survival after thrombotic stroke. (Abstract) *Thromb Haemost* 1979;**42**:161.

27. Gent M, Blakely JA, Hachinski VC, et al. A secondary prevention randomized trial of suloctidil in patients with a recent history of thromboembolic stroke. *Stroke* 1985;**16**:416–424.

28. Swedish Cooperative Study Group. High-dose acetylsalicylic acid after cerebral infarction: a Swedish co-operative study. *Stroke* 1987;**18**:325–334.

29. Gent M, Blakely JA, Easton JD, et al. The Canadian American Ticlopidine Study (CATS) in thromboembolic stroke. *Lancet* 1989;**1**:1215–1220.

30. ESPS Group. European Stroke Prevention Study. *Stroke* 1990;**21**:1122–1130.

31. Elwood PC, Cochrane AL, Burr ML, et al. A randomized controlled trial of acetyl-salicylic acid in the secondary prevention of mortality from myocardial infarction. *Br Med J* 1974;**1**:436–440.

32. The Coronary Drug Project Research Group. Aspirin in coronary heart disease. *J Chronic Dis* 1976;**29**:625–642.

33. Elwood PC, Sweetnam PM. Aspirin and secondary mortality after myocardial infarction. *Lancet* 1979;**2**:1313–1315.

34. Breddin K, Loew D, Lechner K, Uberla K, Walter E. Secondary prevention of myocardial infarction: a comparison of acetylsalicylic acid, placebo and phenprocoumon. *Haemostasis* 1980;**9**:325–344.

35. Aspirin Myocardial Infarction Study Research Group. A randomized, controlled trial of aspirin in persons recovered from myocardial infarction. *JAMA* 1980;**243**:661–669.

36. Persantine-Aspirin Reinfarction Study Research Group. Persantine and aspirin in coronary heart disease. *Circulation* 1980;**62**:449–461.
37. Aspirin after Myocardial Infarction (Editorial). *Lancet* 1980;**1**:1172–1173.
38. ISIS-2 (Second International Study of Infarct Survival) Collaborative Group. Randomised trial of intravenous streptokinase, oral aspirin, both, or neither among 17,187 cases of suspected acute myocardial infarction: ISIS-2. *Lancet* 1988;**2**:349–360.
39. Klimt CR, Knatterud GL, Stamler J, Meier P. Persantine-aspirin reinfarction study. Part II. Secondary coronary prevention with persantine and aspirin. *JACC* 1986;**7**:251–269.
40. Anturane Reinfarction Trial Research Group. Sulfinpyrazone in the prevention of cardiac death after myocardial infarction. The Anturane Reinfarction Trial. *N Engl J Med* 1978;**298**:289–295.
41. Anturane Reinfarction Trial Research Group. Sulfinpyrazone in the prevention of sudden death after myocardial infarction. *N Engl J Med* 1980;**302**:250–256.
42. Temple R, Pledger GW. The FDA's critique of the Anturane Reinfarction Trial. *N Engl J Med* 1980;**303**:1488–1492.
43. Anturane Reinfarction Trial Policy Committee. The Anturane Reinfarction Trial: reevaluation of outcome. *N Engl J Med* 1982;**306**:1005–1008.
44. Gent M. Methodological innovations and controversies: what have we learned from the Anturane Reinfarction Trial? *Progress in Pharmacology* 1982;**4**:51–58.
45. Anturane Reinfarction Italian Study Group. Sulphinpyrazone in post-myocardial infarction. *Lancet* 1982;**1**:237–242.
46. Lewis HD Jr, Davis JW, Archibald DG, et al. Protective effects of aspirin against acute myocardial infarction and death in men with unstable angina: results of a Veterans Administration cooperative study. *N Engl J Med* 1983;**309**:396–403.
47. Cairns JA, Gent M, Singer J, et al. Aspirin, sulfinpyrazone, or both in unstable angina. *N Engl J Med* 1985;**313**:1369–1375.
48. Theroux P, Ouimet H, McCans J, et al. Aspirin, heparin, or both to treat acute unstable angina. *N Engl J Med* 1988;**319**:1105–1111.
49. The RISC Group. Risk of myocardial infarction and death during treatment with low dose aspirin and intravenous heparin in men with unstable coronary artery disease. *Lancet* 1990;**336**:227–230.
50. Balsano F, Rizzon P, Violi F, et al. Antiplatelet treatment with ticlopidine in unstable angina. A controlled multicenter clinical trial. *Circulation* 1990;**82**:17–26.
51. Stiegler H, Hess H, Mietaschk A, Trampisch H-J, Ingrisch H. [The effect of ticlopidine on peripheral obliterative arterial disease]. *Dtsch Med Wochenschr* 1984;**109**:1240–1243.
52. Hess H, Mietaschk A, Deichsel G. Drug-induced inhibition of platelet function delays progression of peripheral occlusive arterial disease. A prospective double-blind arteriographically controlled trial. *Lancet* 1985;**1**:415–419.
53. Boissel JP, Peyrieux JC, Destors JM. Is it possible to reduce the risk of cardiovascular events in subjects suffering from intermittent claudication of the lower limbs? *Thromb Haemost* 1989;**62**:681–685.
54. Janzon L, Bergqvist D, Boberg J, et al. Prevention of myocardial infarction and stroke in patients with intermittent claudication; effects of ticlopidine. Results from STIMS, the Swedish Ticlopidine Multicentre Study. *J Int Med* 1990;**227**:301–308.
55. The Steering Committee of the Physicians' Health Study Research Group. Preliminary report: findings from the aspirin component of the ongoing Physicians' Health Study. *N Engl J Med* 1988;**318**:262–264.

56. The Steering Committee of the Physicians' Health Study Research Group. Final report on the aspirin component of the ongoing Physicians' Health Study. *N Engl J Med* 1989;**321**:129–135.
57. Peto R, Gray R, Collins R, et al. Randomised trial of prophylactic daily aspirin in British male doctors. *Br Med J* 1988;**296**:313–316.
58. Hennekens CH, Peto R, Hutchison GB, Doll R. An overview of the British and American aspirin studies. *N Engl J Med* 1988;**318**:923–924.
59. Antiplatelet Trialists' Collaboration. Secondary prevention of vascular disease by prolonged antiplatelet treatment. *Br Med J* 1988;**296**:320–331.
60. Gent M. Single studies and overview analyses: is aspirin of value in cerebral ischemia? *Stroke* 1987;**18**:541–544.
61. Hirsh J, Salzman EW, Harker L, et al. Aspirin and other platelet active drugs: Relationship among dose, effectiveness and side-effects. *Chest* 1989;**95**(Suppl):12–18.
62. Fuster V, Cohen M, Halperin J. Aspirin in the prevention of coronary disease (Editorial). *N Engl J Med* 1989;**321**:183–185.
63. Roth GJ, Majerus PW. The mechanism of the effect of aspirin on human platelets. 1. Acetylation of a particulate fraction protein. *J Clin Invest* 1975;**56**:624–632.
64. Moncada S, Vane JR. The role of prostacyclin in vascular tissue. *Fed Proc* 1979; **38**:66–71.
65. Levy M. Aspirin use in patients with major upper gastrointestinal bleeding and peptic ulcer. *N Engl J Med* 1974;**290**:1158–1162.

9
An Analysis of the Side Effects of Ticlopidine

BASIL A. MOLONY

Introduction

In this chapter we will review the tolerance and safety of ticlopidine and compare it to that of aspirin, the current standard medication for ischemic stroke prevention, and to placebo treatment. Safety data from our controlled clinical trials on the use of ticlopidine for stroke prevention is quite extensive. Over 4000 patients (approximately 2000 on ticlopidine therapy and 2000 on control therapy) were involved in the combined TASS[1] and CATS[2] trials for durations of up to 5.8 years. Safety data from these double-blind, controlled clinical trials will form this review's primary focus. Extensive postmarketing surveillance (PMS) experience[3] is also available from Europe and Japan to supplement controlled clinical trial data.

Controlled clinical trials can give the essence of a compound's tolerance and safety, but they often exaggerate the true situation. There are a number of reasons for this: heightened sensitivity to body experiences engendered by participation in an investigational drug study; the long litany of possible side effects provided in the informed-consent materials; repeated questioning about adverse experiences at each follow-up visit; and the well-known placebo effect seen in controlled trials.

PMS experience can be even more unreliable in the opposite direction as it often involves under-recognition and under-reporting of safety data. Usually only serious, life-threatening, or fatal adverse reactions are reported, and even these are often gross underestimates. On the other hand, PMS can identify events too rare to be detected in the more limited clinical trials. Even from these extremes of recognition and reporting, however, it is usually possible to derive a balanced account of a drug's side effects and safety profile.

The safety population from the TASS and CATS trials consisted of any patient who took one or more doses of assigned medication. The ticlopidine population consisted of approximately 1500 patients from TASS and 500 patients from CATS (Table 9.1). Because CATS lasted 3 years and TASS lasted almost 6 years, the maximum duration for placebo-treated patients in CATS is less than that for the aspirin- and ticlopidine-treated patients in TASS. On the other hand, the mean duration for ticlopidine-treated patients is less than that

TABLE 9.1. TASS and CATS safety populations, duration on treatment (years).

	N	Mean	Max
Ticlopidine	2048	1.9	5.8
Aspirin	1527	2.4	5.8
Placebo	536	1.6	3.2

for aspirin-treated patients, because it includes the shorter duration of ticlopidine-treated patients in the CATS trial.

Main topics addressed in the safety review are summarized below.
1. *Side effects*. These include any side effects in any therapy group at any time during the 5.8 years of study. It should be noted that these side effects occurred in older individuals who had many coexisting diseases and who were taking many concomitant medications.
2. *Abnormal laboratory values*. These abnormalities lack the subjectivity of patient-reported side effects and provide more objective and tangible data for comparison across treatments. They are also a useful measure of a compound's toxicity.
3. *Hemorrhagic phenomena*. Both ticlopidine and aspirin interfere with the role of platelets in hemostasis and cause prolongation of template bleeding time. Hence, hemorrhagic side effects or complications warrant separate consideration and discussion.
4. *Deaths on study medication*. Therapeutic trials of antiplatelet agents in older individuals involve possible occurrence of stroke, myocardial infarction, and vascular death. It is essential that reductions in these thromboembolic vascular fatalities are not offset by increased fatalities from other causes.
5. *Rare events*. Significant clinical abnormalities are encountered in 1 out of 1000 or more patients exposed to medication. These rare events occasionally surface in therapeutic trials, but they are more likely to be reported in PMS data.
6. *Overdosage*. These data include potential or actual findings attributable to drug overdose.
7. *Contraindications, warnings, and precautions*. These include prohibitions or concerns required by regulatory agencies during use of therapy.

We will conclude with a summary and overview of the relative risks and benefits of ticlopidine vs. currently available therapies.

Side Effects

Any Side Effects

During the trial side effects were reported in 60% of ticlopidine-treated patients and 53% of aspirin-treated patients (Table 9.2). At first glance, these rates seem

TABLE 9.2. Side effects.

	Ticlopidine (%)	Aspirin (%)	Placebo (%)
Any side effect	60	53.2	34.3
Diarrhea	20.7	9.8	10.3
Nausea	11.4	10.2	5.8
Dyspepsia	10.4	13.8	2.1
GI pains	6.9	10.0	4.1
Vomiting	4.0	3.0	2.8
Flatulence	2.4	2.6	0
Anorexia	2.2	1.3	0.4
Rash	11.6	5.2	6.9
Pruritus	3.3	1.2	1.3
Dizziness	3.4	3.0	0.4
Headache	3.1	3.2	1.1
Purpura	3.3	2.4	0.9
Leukopenia	2.4	0.4	1.5
Asthenia	3.6	2.6	0.6

very high. However, it should be remembered that these rates refer to any reported side effects, drug-related or not, in elderly individuals who had many associated diseases. These patients were usually taking multiple drugs and were observed for almost 6 years. The placebo rate of 34% is considerably lower than that of the active drugs. Note, however, that this rate reflects 3 years of experience in CATS vs. almost 6 years of experience in TASS for the two active compounds. As will be discussed later, similar high, side-effect rates have been reported in other trials with similar durations and patient populations.

Most Frequent Side Effects

When summarizing side effects, it is necessary to translate verbatim descriptions into "preferred" terms—realizing that some descriptive nuances are lost in translation. For example, the "preferred" term diarrhea includes various verbatim descriptions such as "loose stools," "frequent bowel movements," etc. This discussion will be limited to the most frequently reported side effects (defined here as side effects occurring in 2% or more of ticlopidine-treated patients).

The most frequent side effects occurred in the digestive system. Diarrhea was the most common side effect, reported by approximately one-fifth of ticlopidine-treated patients. Surprisingly, diarrhea was also frequently reported by aspirin- and placebo-treated patients. There was slightly more nausea, vomiting, and anorexia reported by ticlopidine-treated patients compared to aspirin-treated patients. On the other hand, dyspepsia and gastrointestinal (GI) pains were more frequently reported in aspirin-treated patients. Flatulence was reported equally in ticlopidine- and aspirin-treated patients. In summary, diarrhea was more

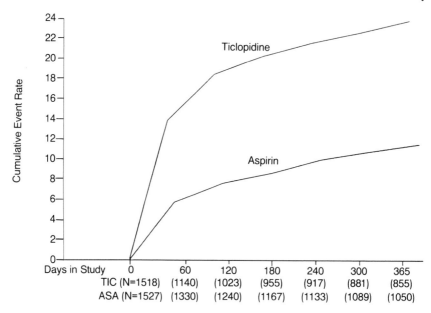

FIGURE 9.1. Side effects: time to onset of diarrhea. Note: N indicates total number of patients
followed up through each time point.

common in ticlopidine-treated patients, whereas indigestion (dyspepsia) and GI
pains were more common in aspirin-treated patients.

The side effect next in frequency in ticlopidine-treated patients was rash. It
was more frequently reported in ticlopidine- than in aspirin- and placebo-treated
patients. The higher rate reported for ticlopidine-treated patients compared to
that for control patients probably represents true ticlopidine-related rashes. These
rashes were usually morbilliform in nature and occasionally urticarial in type.
In general, these occurred during the first 2 months on medication. Thereafter,
rashes were reported with equal frequency in all treatment groups. They were
often associated with pruritus, but occasionally pruritus was reported without
associated rash. Most rashes in control patients consisted of common rashes seen
in routine practice, such as heat rashes, contact dermatitis, and viral exanthemata.

Dizziness and headache were reported with equal frequency by patients
receiving both active treatments.

Purpura, which does not include petechiae, is an interesting side effect because
it can signal vascular dysfunction, thrombocytopenia, or effects of platelet
inhibition. That the purpura observed may sometimes represent "senile" purpura
is suggested by an incidence of almost 1% in placebo treated patients. Purpura
incidence in aspirin treated patients suggests that it is rarely due to thrombocy-

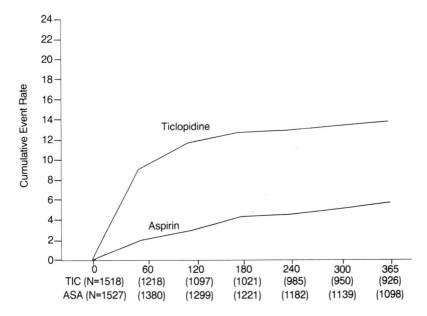

FIGURE 9.2. Side effects: time to onset of rash or urticaria. Note: N indicates total number of patients followed up through each time point.

topenia, because thrombocytopenia is rarely seen in patients on aspirin. This observation is confirmed by platelet count data, presented later in this chapter. The probability that purpura is often caused by platelet function inhibition is supported by the higher incidences of this side effect in treatment groups where platelet function was inhibited. Therapy was rarely discontinued because of purpura, and this side effect was rarely reported as severe.

Occurrences of leukopenia usually consisted of neutropenia. The reported frequency of leukopenia was highest in patients treated with ticlopidine, next highest with aspirin and lowest with placebo. Leukopenia occurrences will not be discussed at this juncture but will be addressed later in the section, "Abnormal Laboratory Values."

Timing of Side Effects

As shown in Figures 9.1 and 9.2, the most frequent and characteristic side effects of ticlopidine tend to occur early in therapy, often beginning after one or a few doses for diarrhea or between 10 to 20 days for rash. Most ticlopidine-related side effects occurred within 2 to 3 months, and premature withdrawals because of side effects usually occurred within the first 3 treatment months. Thereafter, side effects were uncommon and of equal frequency in all three treatment groups.

TABLE 9.3. Premature withdrawals due to side effects (1% or greater in ticlopidine patients).

	Ticlopidine (%) (n = 2048)	Aspirin (%) (n = 1527)	Placebo (%) (n = 536)
% withdrawals for side effects	20.9	14.5	6.7
Diarrhea	6.3	1.8	1.7
Rash	3.4	0.8	0.9
Nausea	2.6	1.9	0.9
GI pain	1.9	2.7	0.4
Leukopenia	1.8	0.2	0.7
Vomiting	1.4	0.9	0.4
Dyspepsia	1.1	2.0	0.2
Abnormal LFTs	1.1	0.3	0.2

Severity

Severity can be categorized either subjectively by the patient or objectively by measurable criteria. For the present review, subjective criteria were accepted.

Of GI system complaints, 9% of ticlopidine-treated patients felt their side effects were severe, compared with 8.7% of aspirin-treated patients. Diarrhea was reported as severe in 4.8% of ticlopidine-treated and 1.9% of aspirin-treated patients. Notable between-treatment differences were evidenced for dyspepsia (0.9% in ticlopidine-treated and 1.8% in aspirin-treated patients) and for GI pain (1.4% ticlopidine and 2.2% aspirin). Otherwise, GI side-effects were reported as equally severe in both groups.

For other body systems, rashes were reported as severe in 2.6% of ticlopidine-treated vs. 0.7% of aspirin-treated patients. Urticaria was reported as severe in 0.6% and 0% of ticlopidine- and aspirin-treated patients, respectively.

With the exception of leukopenia, other severe side effects were rare, and their incidence was similar for the two active compounds.

Outcome

Most side effects were mild, transient, and reversible. Occasionally, especially for diarrhea, transient reduction, or interruption of the ticlopidine dosage schedule was successful in solving the problem. Not all rashes required discontinuation of therapy. Some milder rashes cleared up either spontaneously or while on antihistamine therapy. Other outcomes included discontinuation of therapy or fatalities. Discontinuation rates for the most frequent side effects are shown in Table 9.3. For ticlopidine, discontinuations were most frequent for diarrhea, rash, nausea, and vomiting, while for aspirin, discontinuations were most frequent for dyspepsia and GI pain.

Three fatalities were identified as either directly or indirectly related to the assigned study drugs. One fatality was indirectly related to ticlopidine therapy. This case involved an absolute neutropenia due to ticlopidine therapy, which was associated with septicemia and treated with Tobramycin. The latter drug caused renal toxicity, which was fatal many days after the patient's white count returned to normal.

Two aspirin-related, fatal GI hemorrhages occurred during the trial, although not during the double-blind phase. The two patients were randomized to aspirin but discontinued their double-blind aspirin therapy. They both had fatal GI hemorrhages on open-label aspirin during the follow-up phase of the trial.

Management

Mild side effects or laboratory abnormalities resolved while therapy was continued. Moderate side effects often responded to either temporary reductions or interruptions of therapy or, occasionally, to symptomatic therapy. Severe side effects, or progressions to severe side effects, rarely responded to symptomatic therapies or dosage reductions; therapy had to be discontinued. These side effects resolved rapidly when ticlopidine was discontinued.

Abnormal Laboratory Values

Safety, as distinct from tolerance, was monitored by various laboratory tests. Complete blood counts (CBCs), urinalyses, and biochemical profiles were performed at a central laboratory and measured at baseline, month 1, month 4, and every 4 months thereafter for the balance of the study. In addition, because of reports of neutropenia during the trial's planning stages, monitoring for ticlopidine-related neutropenia was instituted as part of the study design. CBCs, including platelet counts, were performed locally by the investigator at baseline, every 2 weeks for the initial 3 months, monthly until month 6, and every 4 months from month 8 onward.

Results of these local and central laboratory tests formed the laboratory database for detection and follow-up of safety issues associated with drug use. Laboratory abnormalities were detected by two analyses: 1) mean and median values and other standard statistical parameters; and 2) threshold values that were preselected to detect and document possible pathology. These threshold values were specially chosen to be either above or below normal ranges for these tests and, consequently, more likely to reflect actual abnormalities.

Urinalysis data failed to show any significant or consistent abnormalities in any of the treatment groups. CBC values showed changes in mean values and threshold values as follows: mean white blood cell (WBC), neutrophil and lymphocyte counts tended to be lower in ticlopidine-treated patients than in aspirin- or placebo-treated patients. The decreased values were most common at months 1 and 4 and less common at later visits, when they approached control values. The extent of these mean decreases at month 1, the time of greatest reduction for all tests, ranged from 10% to 11% for neutrophil and WBC counts, respectively, to 14% for lymphocyte counts.

Threshold values preselected to detect neutropenia were as follows:

1. *Mild neutropenia* was defined as an absolute neutrophil count (ANC) between 801 and 1200 ANC/mm^3. When ANC values fell into this range, a repeat CBC was required every 2 days until ANC values increased above 1200 or dropped below 800. Therapy did not need to be discontinued for mild neutropenia.
2. *Moderate neutropenia* was defined as an ANC between 451 and 800/mm^3. Therapy did not need to be discontinued, but CBCs were required daily until recovery (ANC 1200/mm^3) or until ANC values decreased below 450/mm^3.
3. *Severe neutropenia* was defined as an ANC of less than or equal to 450/mm^3. It required immediate and permanent discontinuation of therapy and daily CBCs until ANC values increased above 1200/mm^3. Table 9.4 shows the results of this monitoring program.

Severe neutropenia, which was usually considered to be definitely drug-related, occurred in 0.8% of ticlopidine-treated patients. One patient (0.2%) on placebo therapy was receiving a combination of two drugs known to have potential for neutropenia. Severe neutropenia cases due to ticlopidine occurred between days 26 and 62 of study drug therapy. In six of the 17 patients ANC values reached zero. Therapy was discontinued—as mandated—in all 17 severe cases, and recovery occurred in all cases. The time to recovery, defined as ANC values > 1200/mm^3, ranged from 4 to 21 days with a mean duration of 13 days. In one patient, a serious systemic infection occurred. As previously described, this patient's neutropenia abated in approximately 3 weeks, but the patient subsequently died of renal toxicity associated with antibiotic therapy.

Moderate neutropenia occurred in 0.2% of ticlopidine-treated patients. Discontinuation of therapy was not required, but therapy was locally discontinued in two of the four patients. Recovery rate was equally rapid whether or not therapy was discontinued.

Mild neutropenia occurred in all three treatment groups throughout the study, even at screening, and it was more frequent in black patients. Recurrent mild neutropenia of an idiopathic nature, unrelated to drug therapy or disease states, often occurs in blacks. This situation may present some difficulties in utilizing therapy in an intelligent and safe manner. No cases of severe neutropenia occurred in black patients. As with moderate neutropenia, investigators decided to discontinue therapy in approximately one-third of the mild cases. Recovery was rapid and complete whether or not therapy was discontinued. Prevalence of mild neutropenia in ticlopidine-treated patients is probably related to the drug and may resemble the transient mild cases seen on other drugs such as phenothiazine.[4]

On the basis of data from these controlled clinical trials, supplemented by data from PMS studies, various drug regulatory agencies are recommending that

TABLE 9.4. TASS and CATS—neutropenia.

	Ticlopidine (n = 2043)	Aspirin (n = 1527)	Placebo (n = 536)
ANC 800–1200	29 (1.4%)	12 (0.8%)	4 (0.7%)
ANC 451–800	4 (0.2%)	0 (0.0%)	1 (0.2%)
ANC 0–450	17 (0.8%)	0 (0.0%)	1 (0.2%)

CBCs be measured every 2 weeks for the initial 3 months on ticlopidine therapy and that therapy be discontinued when ANC values decrease below 1200/mm^3. After 3 months, CBC measurements should be considered for patients with signs or symptoms of infection. More frequent monitoring during the initial 3 months should also be considered if there is an infection or if the most recent ANC has shown evidence of rapid decline.

Thrombocytopenia has rarely been reported in PMS data. In TASS and CATS, the incidence of mild thrombocytopenia (60,000–80,000 platelets/mm^3) was equal in all three treatment groups. One documented case of severe thrombocytopenia (< 40,000 platelets/mm^3) occurred in a ticlopidine-treated patient. This patient had a typical clinical picture of thrombotic thrombocytopenic purpura (TTP) and responded satisfactorily to plasmapheresis therapy. TTP will be discussed later in the "Rare Events" section.

Changes in biochemistry values were of two kinds: 1) changes in mean values, and 2) abnormal values in individual patients. Changes in mean values will be presented first. Individual test abnormalities will be discussed later in this section, using threshold values to detect possible or actual organ pathology while on therapy or due to therapy.

There were basically no changes in ticlopidine-treated patients compared to aspirin- and placebo-treated patients over time for the following blood chemistry tests: calcium, phosphorus, glucose, total protein, albumin, and globulin, direct bilirubin, and lactic dehydrogenase (LDH). The following tests showed a decrease while on therapy: blood urea nitrogen (BUN)—a reduction of around 6% in the ticlopidine and placebo groups; uric acid—about a 12% decrease in males and females in the ticlopidine group; total bilirubin—the greatest reduction of about 20% at 1 month, but decreased values persisting as long as ticlopidine therapy was continued; and serum glutamic oxaloacetic transaminase (SGOT)— a gradual decrease in all three treatment groups, with a 31% decrease in the ticlopidine group and a 16% decrease in the aspirin and placebo groups, all maximal in the second treatment year.

On the other hand, some mean values increased as follows: creatinine—in ticlopidine-treated patients, an increase of about 5% at 1 month but less thereafter; alkaline phosphatase—in ticlopidine patients only, with the maximal increase of 15% at 1 month, which persisted as long as therapy was continued; total iron—in ticlopidine patients an 18% increase, maximal at 8 months; and gamma glutamyl transpeptidase (GGTP)—a 64% increase at 1 month in ticlopidine patients, with a gradual reduction to normal thereafter. Many of these enzyme changes would seem to be consistent with ticlopidine-related enzyme induction or inhibition.

One test of particular interest and concern was an increase of about 10% in total serum cholesterol in ticlopidine-treated patients. This change was in evidence at month 1 and maximal at month 4, with no further increases thereafter. The reason for this increase (increased absorption, increased production, or decreased removal of cholesterol) is unknown. The last reason is perhaps most likely, but this conclusion is based on limited supporting information. This question is currently being studied. When the unblinded safety committee for these trials learned that cholesterol values were increased, it requested that one-time lipoprotein fractionation profiles be obtained on all active patients.

An analysis of the lipoprotein subtypes (HDL cholesterol, LDL cholesterol, and VLDL cholesterol) showed that all lipoprotein fractions increased almost proportionately. Serum triglycerides and serum cholesterol were also increased in ticlopidine-treated patients, and this finding would account for the increase in VLDL cholesterol. Ratios of HDL cholesterol to atherogenic cholesterol (LDL-C) and total cholesterol were the same in all three treatment groups, which may help to explain the lower vascular thrombosis rates in ticlopidine-treated patients compared with aspirin-treated patients in TASS and placebo-treated patients in CATS.

Threshold Values

Threshold or clinical decision-level values were selected for analysis before study unblinding. These values were based on both literature values[5] and personal experience with various disease markers. The following tests revealed clinically significant abnormalities while on therapies:

1. *Total bilirubin.* Two threshold levels of bilirubin were selected for review: > 2.0 mg/dl and >2.5 mg/dl. Total bilirubin values of >2.0 mg/dl did not seem to be diagnostic of clinical jaundice, since more elevations of this magnitude were seen in placebo-treated patients than in those receiving active drugs. Total bilirubin values of >2.5 mg, a threshold value usually selected to define clinical jaundice, correlated well with clinical diagnoses of jaundice made by attending physicians. Using the latter as a threshold value, there were two aspirin-treated patients with jaundice. In one of the aspirin-treated patients, jaundice was associated with congestive heart failure that was subsequently fatal. Direct bilirubin values were normal in this patient. In the second patient, a data transcription error accounted for the abnormal value.

There were 6 ticlopidine-treated patients with total bilirubin values of >2.5 mg/dl. One value was associated with acute cholecystitis with biliary calculi; a second with congestive heart failure; a third with complex medical illness (the jaundice cleared up during therapy when these illnesses were clinically corrected); and a fourth with multiple laboratory abnormalities on day 1410 of the

TABLE 9.5. Abnormal SGOT (combined TASS and CATS data).

Test	Ticlopidine (1072 pts)	Aspirin (1295 pts)	Placebo (453 pts)
SGOT > 100 μ/ml	52 (3.1%)	27 (2.1%)	18 (4.0%)
SGOT > 200 μ/ml	14 (0.8%)	7 (0.5%)	4 (0.9%)
SGOT > 300 μ/ml	10 (0.6%)	6 (0.5%)	2 (0.4%)
SGOT > 400 μ/ml	1 (0.06%)	1 (0.08%)	1 (0.2%)

study. In the last case, repeat values taken within 1 week were normal; the study center blamed a poor lab specimen for the multiple abnormalities. In the two remaining patients, ticlopidine-induced cholestatic jaundice was diagnosed. In one patient there was a serum bilirubin of 6.9 mg/dl on day 27, and in another, a total bilirubin of 4.2 mg/dl on day 55. Supporting tests (including direct bilirubin, alkaline phosphatase, serum cholesterol, and urinalysis) were also consistent with cholestatic jaundice. The clinical picture reversed rapidly when therapy was discontinued. The only observation of note in these two patients was a concomitant use of sulfonylurea drugs for maturity onset diabetes.

2. *SGOT values.* Various threshold levels for SGOT (normal range 5–50 μ/ml) values were selected for review. As Table 9.5 shows, elevations were equally frequent in all three treatment groups. Each patient's data was reviewed, and there was no evidence of drug hepatitis. Most elevations were transient and isolated, and they resolved while on therapy. In some cases, there were obvious explanations—such as ethanol abuse, viral hepatitis, or congestive heart failure. A review of all other tests employing the preselected threshold values failed to identify evidence of target-organ damage or toxicity related to study medications.

Hemorrhagic Phenomena

Because ticlopidine and aspirin inhibit platelet function and prolong bleeding time, there is a possibility of increased bleeding tendency. Three subcategories of bleeding manifestations were examined: generalized hemorrhagic events, gastrointestinal hemorrhage, and intracranial hemorrhage.

Generalized Hemorrhagic Events

These events were reported by 8.3% of ticlopidine-treated patients, 10.0% of aspirin-treated patients and 3.0% of placebo-treated patients. The most frequent of these events were purpura (3.3% ticlopidine, 2.4% aspirin), epistaxis (1.9% ticlopidine, 2.2% aspirin), hematuria (0.7% ticlopidine, 1.2% aspirin), and petechiae (0.2% in both ticlopidine and aspirin). Other generalized hemorrhagic events were even more rare.

Gastrointestinal Hemorrhage

Because of aspirin's propensity to cause upper GI bleeding, an examination of upper GI bleeding and occurrence of peptic ulceration was undertaken in all three treatment groups. Upper GI bleeding in the three patient groups was reported as 1.5% for ticlopidine, 3.1% for aspirin, and 0.6% for placebo. Peptic ulceration was diagnosed in 0.6% of the ticlopidine group, 2.9% of the aspirin group, and 0.0% of the placebo group. Furthermore, termination of study medication for serious GI hemorrhage occurred in 0.5% of ticlopidine-treated, 1.6% of aspirin-treated, and 0.2% of placebo-treated patients. Termination of study drugs for peptic ulceration was 0.05% for ticlopidine, 1.2% for aspirin, and 0% for placebo. In the TASS trial, which involved a direct comparison of aspirin with ticlopidine, 16 aspirin-treated patients were hospitalized for GI bleeding. Twelve of the 16 required a blood transfusion. Only one ticlopidine-treated patient required hospitalization; that patient was also transfused.

Intracranial Hemorrhage

In TASS, out of a total of 128 strokes while on ticlopidine and 198 while on aspirin, only five were associated with intracerebral hemorrhages while on ticlopidine and six while on aspirin. There was one hemorrhagic infarction while on ticlopidine and three while on aspirin. In addition, there was one nonfatal subarachnoid hemorrhage while on ticlopidine and none while on aspirin. In CATS, there were no hemorrhagic infarctions while on ticlopidine and two while on placebo. There was one cerebral hemorrhage (fatal) while on ticlopidine and none on placebo. For subarachnoid hemorrhage, the numbers were zero for ticlopidine and two for placebo. Data on intracranial hemorrhages do not suggest any greater occurrence of these events in these studies. They also do not suggest any increased occurrences while on antiplatelet drugs compared with placebo or while on ticlopidine compared with aspirin.

Deaths on Study Medication

Figure 9.3 illustrates deaths occurring while on study medication and within 10 days of discontinuing study drugs in both the TASS and CATS trials. Because the present review's focus is on safety endpoints, only patients who took at least one dose of study drug are counted in these analyses. A 10-day safety rule was adopted for all side effects before unblinding of the trials and was chosen for a number of biological reasons: 1) life span of a platelet is approximately 10 days; 2) reversal of the study drug's antiplatelet effect takes approximately 10 days after discontinuation of therapy; 3) clearance of substantial amounts of ticlopidine from the body takes about 10 days; 4) proper accounting for deaths that occurred within 10 days of stopping therapy but may have been related to therapy.

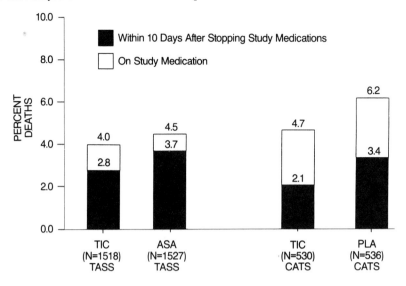

FIGURE 9.3. Ticlopidine safety death.

A review of the deaths occurring while on therapy shows that the fatality rate was always less while on ticlopidine than on control therapy. If the 10-day rule is used, fatality rates were still lower while on ticlopidine. These data include deaths from all causes and therefore include stroke deaths, cardiac deaths, medical illness-related deaths, surgical deaths, cancer deaths, and deaths from trauma.

A review of the various individual causes of death failed to show any category in which ticlopidine mortality rates exceeded control rates. Ticlopidine rates were usually lower and occasionally equal to control rates. It was reassuring to discover that deaths from strokes or other thrombotic events were not offset by increases in deaths from other causes. The higher overall mortality rates in CATS patients compared to TASS patients, who were studied for twice the duration of CATS patients, probably reflect the fact that CATS patients were older and sicker than TASS patients.

Rare Events

Rare events are occasionally reported during clinical trials while patients are taking study medication or in PMS data while patients are on therapy, but circumstances may suggest that these events are related to therapy. Often the timing, frequency, and evolution of the event make attribution to the drug likely or certain. When there is an isolated occurrence and no other explanation is forthcoming, attribution must be presumed even though it can't be proved.

Rechallenge is often not possible or defensible. The following rare but serious side effects or illnesses have occurred in ticlopidine-treated patients.

Pancytopenia. This side effect has been reported from PMS monitoring. In some cases the myelogram and/or bone marrow biopsy have shown the depression of all three cell lines, or in extreme cases, a picture of bone marrow aplasia (aplastic anemia). Frequency, timing, and evolution of the events in question make attribution to therapy obvious. If detected early with routine CBC monitoring and if therapy is discontinued, there is usually prompt recovery.

Hemolytic Anemia with Associated Reticulocytosis. Only a few cases have been reported, but attribution to ticlopidine seems fairly definite.

Allergic Pneumonitis in Association with Acute Neuropathy. This side effect was reported in a single patient in the TASS trial. As described clinically and by biopsy, the allergic pneumonitis was reminiscent of that seen with other drugs, such as nitrofurantoin. The timing, evolution, and resolution of both side effects make attribution to ticlopidine very likely. No rechallenge was undertaken.

Systemic Lupus Erythematosus (SLE). An association between ticlopidine use and SLE is unclear but possible. In controlled clinical trials, including the STIMS trial,[5] evidence of SLE was reported with almost equal frequency in control patients as in ticlopidine patients. The PMS experience is not of value in addressing this question.

Vasculitis, Serum Sickness Arthropathy, and Myositis. A few cases of each of these illnesses have been reported. Their relationship to therapy seems possible.

Hepatitis. Cases of hepatitis related to ticlopidine have been reported in the PMS program, and its attribution to the therapy appears likely.

Cholestatic Jaundice. This side effect has been identified in controlled clinical trials and has also been reported in PMS data. A cause-and-effect relationship seems definite.

Nephrotic Syndrome. The one reported episode (TASS) was of a 70-year-old patient who was normal at enrollment. He had had a nephrectomy 8 years previously for hypernephroma. After 1 month on ticlopidine therapy, he had marked edema and heavy albuminuria. His nephrologist diagnosed nephrotic syndrome. Ticlopidine was discontinued, and the albuminuria cleared up within 1 month.

Hyponatremia. This side effect occurred while on ticlopidine in TASS, but attribution is questionable because there was a further recurrence approximately $2\frac{1}{2}$ months after ticlopidine was discontinued.

Immune Thrombocytopenic Purpura. This side effect has rarely been identified, either in controlled clinical trials or in PMS surveys.

Thrombotic Thrombocytopenia Purpura (TTP). The first and only case of TTP while on ticlopidine in a controlled clinical trial occurred in 1983, and the patient responded completely to plasmapheresis. This was the only case among the approximately 3000 ticlopidine-treated patients in all of the therapeutic trials in North America. Since that time, additional cases have been reported in the PMS database. Four of these cases have been published.[7]

A review of available data suggests that TTP is a rare side effect of ticlopidine. Present evidence relates to the usual timing of this event after initiation of therapy. Onset of TTP is usually within 60 days of starting ticlopidine. Additional information regarding TTP shows that the event can occur at any age and in females as well as males. Fatalities can occur, however, a fatal outcome is very unlikely if patients are treated early and aggressively with plasmapheresis. Favorable outcomes with plasmapheresis therapy are in line with recently published data on the effectiveness of plasmapheresis for TTP vs. other treatment modalities.[8]

Overdosage

Only one case of deliberate overdosage with ticlopidine has been reported from the foreign PMS database. It involved ingestion of a single 6000 mg dose of ticlopidine (or 24 standard 250 mg tablets). The only reported abnormalities were prolongation of bleeding time and increased serum glutamic pyruvic transaminase (SGPT) values. No special therapy was instituted, and the patient recovered without sequelae.

Although not reported in the above case, one might also expect such GI symptoms as nausea, vomiting, abdominal cramps, and diarrhea with overdosage because of the frequency of these types of side effects with standard doses of ticlopidine.

Contraindications, Warnings, and Precautions

Contraindications

Individual contraindications included in the current U.S.-approved label are as follows (quoted verbatim):

- Hypersensitivity to the drug.
- Presence of hematopoietic disorders such as neutropenia and thrombocytopenia.
  [*Comment.* We have no experience with the use of ticlopidine in patients with these disorders. We don't know if patients with preexisting neutropenia are at additional or increased risk for ticlopidine-induced neutropenia—so this is a rational contraindication. Ticlopidine rarely causes thrombocytopenia on its own. However, it would be unwise and potentially unsafe to inhibit platelet function when platelet numbers are already low.]
- Presence of a hemostatic disorder or active pathological bleeding (such as bleeding peptic ulcer or intracranial bleeding).
  [*Comment.* Again, it would be unwise and potentially unsafe to inhibit platelet function and prolong bleeding time in the presence of clinically worrisome bleeding situations.]

- Patients with severe liver impairment.

  [*Comment*. Ticlopidine is metabolized by the liver. Additionally, in cases of advanced liver impairment, coagulation factors may not be produced in adequate amounts, or portal hypertension with varices may be present. These conditions could greatly increase the risk of hemorrhage.]

Warnings

These issues have been addressed in other sections of this chapter, but these warnings from the approved label for ticlopidine bear repeating. They are reproduced verbatim as follows:

WARNINGS

Neutropenia

Neutropenia defined in these studies as an ANC < 1200 neutrophils/mm^3 occurred in 50 of 2,048 (2.4%) stroke patients who received TICLID in clinical trials.

Severe Neutropenia (<450 neutrophils/mm^3):

Severe neutropenia and/or agranulocytosis occurred in 17 of the 2048 (0.8%) patients who received TICLID. When the drug was discontinued in these patients, the neutrophil counts returned to normal (> 1200 neutrophils/mm^3) within 1–3 weeks.

Mild to Moderate Neutropenia (451–1200 neutrophils/mm^3):

Mild to moderate neutropenia occurred in 33 of the 2048 (1.6%) patients who received TICLID. Eleven of the patients discontinued treatment and recovered within a few days. In the remaining 22 patients, the neutropenia was transient and did not require discontinuation of therapy.

The onset of severe neutropenia occurred 3 weeks to 3 months after the start of therapy with TICLID, with no documented cases of severe neutropenia beyond that time in the large controlled trials. The bone marrow typically showed a reduction in myeloid precursors.

It is therefore essential that CBCs and white cell differentials be performed every two weeks starting from the second week to the end of the third month of therapy with TICLID, but more frequent monitoring is necessary for patients whose absolute neutrophil counts have been consistently declining or are 30% less than the baseline count.

Neutropenia (an absolute neutrophil count (ANC) of less than 1200 neutrophils/mm^3) is calculated as follows: ANC = WBC × %neutrophils. If clinical evaluation and repeat laboratory testing confirm the presence of neutropenia (< 1200/mm^3), the drug should be discontinued.

In clinical trials, when therapy was discontinued immediately upon detection of neutropenia, the neutrophil counts returned to normal within 1–3 weeks.

After the first three months of therapy, CBCs need be obtained only for patients with signs or symptoms suggestive of infection.

Thrombocytopenia

Rarely, thrombocytopenia may occur in isolation or together with neutropenia.

If clinical evaluation and repeat laboratory testing confirm the presence of thrombocytopenia ($< 80,000$ cells/mm^3), the drug should be discontinued.

Cholesterol Elevation

TICLID$^®$ therapy causes increased serum cholesterol and triglycerides. Serum total cholesterol levels are increased 8–10% within one month of therapy and persist at that level. The ratios of the lipoprotein subfractions are unchanged.

Other Hematological Effects

Rare cases of pancytopenia and thrombotic thrombocytopenic purpura, some of which have been fatal, have been reported in Post-Marketing Surveillance.

Anticoagulant Drugs

The tolerance and safety of coadministration of TICLID with heparin, oral anticoagulants, or fibrinolytic agents has not been established. If a patient is switched from an anticoagulant or fibrinolytic drug to TICLID, the former drug should be discontinued prior to TICLID administration.

Precautions

The precautions from the U.S.-approved label are quoted verbatim:

General

TICLID should be used with caution in patients who may be at risk of increased bleeding from trauma, surgery, or pathological conditions. If it is desired to eliminate the antiplatelet effects of TICLID prior to elective surgery, the drug should be discontinued 10–14 days prior to surgery. Several controlled clinical studies have found increased surgical blood loss in patients undergoing surgery during treatment with ticlopidine. In TASS and CATS it was recommended that patients have ticlopidine discontinued prior to elective surgery. Several hundred patients underwent surgery during the trials, and no excessive surgical bleeding was reported.

Prolonged bleeding time is normalized within two hours after administration of 20 mg methylprednisolone i.v. Platelet transfusions may also be used to reverse the effect of TICLID on bleeding.

GI Bleeding

TICLID prolongs template bleeding time. The drug should be used with caution in patients who have lesions with a propensity to bleed (such as ulcers). Drugs that might induce such lesions should be used with caution in patients on TICLID. (See Contraindications.)

Use in Hepatically Impaired Patients

Because of limited experience in patients with severe hepatic disease, who may have bleeding diatheses, the use of TICLID is not recommended in this population. (See Clinical Pharmacology and Contraindications.)

Use in Renally Impaired Patients

There is limited experience in patients with renal impairment. In controlled clinical trials, no unexpected problems have been encountered in patients having mild renal impairment and there is no experience with dosage adjustment in patients with greater degrees of renal impairment. Nevertheless, for renally impaired patients it may be necessary to reduce the dosage of ticlopidine or discontinue it altogether, if hemorrhagic or hematopoietic problems are encountered. (See Clinical Pharmacology.)

Information for the Patient (See PPI)

Patients should be told that a decrease in the number of white blood cells (neutropenia) can occur with TICLID®, especially during the first three months of treatment, and that if neutropenia is severe, it could result in an increased risk of infection. They should be told it is critically important to obtain the scheduled blood tests to detect neutropenia. Patients should also be reminded to contact their physicians if they experience any indication of infection such as fever, chills, and sore throat, all of which may be consequences of neutropenia.

All patients should be told that it may take them longer than usual to stop bleeding when they take TICLID and that they should report any unusual bleeding to their physician. Patients should tell physicians and dentists that they are taking TICLID before any surgery is scheduled and before any new drug is prescribed.

Patients should be told to report promptly side effects of TICLID such as severe or persistent diarrhea, skin rashes, or subcutaneous bleeding, or any signs of cholestasis, such as yellow skin or sclera, dark urine, or light colored stools.

Patients should be told to take TICLID with food or just after eating in order to minimize gastrointestinal discomfort.

Laboratory Tests

Liver Function: TICLID therapy has been associated with elevations of alkaline phosphatase and transaminases which generally occurred within 1–4 months of therapy initiation. In controlled clinical trials, the incidence of elevated alkaline phosphatase (greater than 2 times upper limit of normal) was 7.6% in ticlopidine patients, 6.0% in placebo patients, and 2.5% in aspirin patients. The incidence of elevated AST (SGOT) (greater than 2 times upper limit of normal) was 3.1% in ticlopidine patients, 4.0% in placebo patients, and 2.1% in aspirin patients. No progressive increases were observed in closely monitored clinical trials (e.g. no transaminase greater than 10 times the upper limit of normal was seen), but most patients with these abnormalities had therapy discontinued. Occasionally patients had developed minor elevations in bilirubin.

Based on post-marketing and clinical trials experiences, liver function testing should be considered whenever liver dysfunction is suspected, particularly during the first four months of treatment.

Drug Interactions

Therapeutic doses of TICLID caused a 30% increase in the plasma half-life of antipyrine and may cause analogous effects on similarly metabolized drugs. Therefore the dose of drugs metabolized by hepatic microsomal enzymes with low therapeutic ratios, or being given to patients with hepatic impairment, may require adjustment to maintain optimal therapeutic blood levels when starting or stopping concomitant therapy with ticlopidine. Studies of specific drug interactions yielded the following results:

Aspirin: Aspirin did not modify the ticlopidine-mediated inhibition of ADP-induced platelet aggregation, but ticlopidine potentiated the effect of aspirin on collagen-induced platelet aggregation. The safety of this combination has not been established, and concomitant use of aspirin and ticlopidine is not recommended. (See Precautions—GI Bleeding).

Antacids: Administration of TICLID after antacids resulted in an 18% decrease in plasma levels of ticlopidine.

Cimetidine: Chronic administration of cimetidine reduced the clearance of a single dose of TICLID by 50%.

Digoxin: Co-administration of TICLID with digoxin resulted in a slight decrease (approximately 15%) in digoxin plasma levels. Little or no change in therapeutic efficacy of digoxin would be expected.

Theophylline: In normal volunteers, concomitant administration of TICLID resulted in a significant increase in the theophylline elimination half-life from 8.6 to 12.2 hr and a comparable reduction in total plasma clearance of theophylline.

Phenobarbital: In six normal volunteers, the inhibitory effects of TICLID on platelet aggregation were not altered by chronic administration of phenobarbital.

Phenytoin: In vitro studies demonstrated that ticlopidine does not alter the plasma protein binding of phenytoin. However, the protein binding interactions of ticlopidine and its metabolites have not been studied in vivo. Caution should be exercised in coadministering this drug with TICLID, and it may be useful to remeasure phenytoin blood concentrations.

Propranolol: In vitro studies demonstrated that ticlopidine does not alter the plasma protein binding of propranolol. However, the protein binding interactions of ticlopidine and its metabolites have not been studied in vivo. Caution should be exercised in coadministering this drug with TICLID.

Other Concomitant Therapy: Although specific interaction studies were not performed, in clinical studies, TICLID was used concomitantly with beta blockers, calcium channel blockers, diuretics, and nonsteroidal anti-inflammatory drugs without evidence of clinically significant adverse interactions. (See Precautions.)

Food Interaction: The oral bioavailability of ticlopidine is increased by 20% when taken after a meal. Administration of TICLID with food is recommended to maximize gastrointestinal tolerance. In controlled trials, TICLID was taken with meals.

Carcinogenesis, Mutagenesis, Impairment of Fertility

In a two-year oral carcinogenicity study in rats, ticlopidine at daily doses of up to 100 mg/kg ($610/mg/m^2$) was not tumorigenic. For a 70 kg person ($1.73m^2$ body surface are), the dose represents 14 times the recommended clinical dose on a mg/kg basis and 2 times the clinical dose of body surface area basis. In a 78 week oral carcinogenicity study in mice ticlopidine at daily doses up to 275 mg/kg (1180 mg/m^2) was not tumorigenic. The dose represents 40 times the recommended clinical dose on a mg/kg basis and 4 times the clinical dose on body surface area basis.

Ticlopidine was not mutagenic in *in vitro* Ames test, rat hepatocyte DNA-repair assay, and Chinese hamster fibroblast chromosomal aberration test and *in vivo* mouse spermatozoid morphology test, Chinese hamster micronucleus test, and Chinese hamster bone marrow cell sister chromatid exchange test. Ticlopidine was found to have no effect on fertility of male and female rats on oral doses up to 400 mg/kg/day.

Pregnancy: Teratogenic Effects

Pregnancy Category B. Teratology studies have been conducted in mice (doses up to 200 mg/kg/day), rats (doses up to 400 mg/kg/day), and rabbits (doses up to 200 mg/kg/day). Doses of 400 mg/kg in rats, 200 mg/kg/day in mice, and 100 mg/kg in rabbits produced maternal toxicity as well as fetal toxicity, but there was no evidence of a teratogenic potential of ticlopidine. There are, however, no adequate and well-controlled studies in pregnant women. Because animal reproduction studies are not always predictive of human response, this drug should be used during pregnancy only if clearly needed.

Nursing Mothers

Studies in rats have shown ticlopidine is excreted in the milk. It is not known whether this drug is excreted in human milk. Because many drugs are excreted in human milk and because of the potential for serious adverse reactions in nursing infants from ticlopidine, a decision should be made whether to discontinue nursing or to discontinue the drug, taking into account the importance of the drug to the mother.

Pediatric Use

Safety and efficacy in patients under the age of 18 have not been established.

Geriatric Use

Clearance of ticlopidine is somewhat lower in elderly patients and trough levels are increased. The major clinical trials with TICLID were conducted in an elderly population with an average of 64 years. Of the total number of patients in the therapeutic trials, 45% of patients were over 65 years old and 12% were over 75 years old. No overall differences in effectiveness or safety were observed between these patients and younger patients, and other reported clinical experience has not identified differences in responses between the elderly and younger patients, but greater sensitivity of some older individuals cannot be ruled out.

Summary and Perspective

The safety database on ticlopidine is substantial in amount, duration, and detail, permitting definite conclusions and recommendations for future patients. Incidence of all side effects, as well as individual side effects, seems high. However, these findings are not unusual when compared to other studies with similar patient populations and durations. In the UK-TIA trial, approximately 50% of high-dose (1200 mg daily) aspirin-treated patients, 40% of low-dose (300 mg daily) aspirin-treated patients, and almost 30% of placebo-treated patients reported GI side effects.[9] Information on side effects affecting other body systems was not provided.

A high rate of side effects was also reported in the British Male Doctors Aspirin Prophylaxis Trial.[10] Premature withdrawals for side effects were even higher than in the ticlopidine trials, but the pattern for premature withdrawal was similar. The greatest percentage occurred during year 1

(19.5%) and a lesser percentage during the subsequent 5 years (a total of 24.8% during the 5 years).

Gurwitz and Avorn have considered the question of adverse drug reactions and their relationship to advancing age.[11] They admit that a lack of studies exists addressing this question since many trials exclude elderly subjects. They state that "patient-specific physiologic and functional characteristics are probably more important than any chronologic measure in predicting both adverse and beneficial outcomes associated with specific drug therapies."

Our safety data showed slight increases in total side effects using age 65 as a separation point. For patients under age 65, side-effect rates were as follows: ticlopidine 59.8%, placebo 19.4%, and aspirin 52.3%. For patients aged 65 or older, the rates were: ticlopidine 60.3%, placebo 35.5%, and aspirin 54.4%. However, some individual side effects showed even wider variations. A few examples will suffice. Diarrhea occurred in 18.7% of ticlopidine-treated patients under age 65 vs. 23.1% over age 65. Dyspepsia occurred in 12% of ticlopidine-treated patients under age 65 vs. 8.5% over age 65. Rash occurred in 12.6% of ticlopidine-treated patients under age 65 vs. 10.5% over age 65. In general, placebo-treated patients over age 65 reported more nausea, dyspepsia, GI pains, and rashes than patients under age 65. Among aspirin-treated patients, differences were not pronounced—with only a slightly higher rate of the above-mentioned side effects in those over age 65 compared to those under age 65.

Side effects analyzed by gender showed definitely higher rates in females than in males. An analysis by race showed a lower incidence in nonwhite (mostly black) patients compared to white patients.

Premature withdrawal rates for side effects in ticlopidine-treated patients seem quite high, but withdrawal rates were also high in the aspirin and placebo groups. High rates of premature withdrawal are also reported in other studies. The premature withdrawal rate for the 500 mg daily aspirin dose in the British Male Physicians trial was about 45%.[10]

Concerning toxicity related to ticlopidine, our studies confirm the fact that ticlopidine causes neutropenia. Incidence of severe drug-related neutropenia seems to be around 1%, usually occurring within 3 months of therapy initiation, and is reversible within 3 weeks when therapy is discontinued. Frequent monitoring during the initial 3 months of therapy is essential for achieving timely detection and correction of the problem. This monitoring could prevent septic complications from sustained undetected neutropenia and could also reduce the potential for fatal outcomes. Other manifestations of organ toxicity are rarely encountered. Usually, they are clinically detectable conditions, such as jaundice and thrombocytopenia.

Questions always arise about the relative cost, safety, and efficacy of ticlopidine compared to aspirin. Obviously, ticlopidine or any other newly developed medication cannot compete with aspirin on a cost basis. The safety issue is complex because of the generally perceived tolerance and safety of aspirin. However, this sense of familiarity fails to take into account the great number of people who are hypersensitive or intolerant to aspirin. In addition, most therapeutic trials of aspirin exclude such patients.

Finally, the issue of aspirin's safety in aspirin-tolerant patients must be considered. In TASS, the incidence of severe GI bleeding that required hospitalization and transfusion and of fatal GI bleeding exceeded the rate of serious neutropenia in ticlopidine-treated patients. Data from other studies using lower doses of aspirin—such as the UK-TIA trial, the British Male Doctors Aspirin Prophylactic Trial, the Dutch TIA trial[12] and the SALT trial[13]—all confirm a high incidence of fatal and severe GI and intracranial bleeding. The rates of these life-threatening bleeding events in aspirin-treated patients were either greater than or equal to those potentially life-threatening events identified in ticlopidine-treated patients.

The relative efficacy of ticlopidine compared to aspirin is another vexing question because of uncertainty about both the optimal dose of aspirin and patient types (male vs. female and threatened stroke vs. recurrent stroke) who respond to aspirin. Ticlopidine's efficacy has been addressed in an earlier chapter. This author's assessment of efficacy data focuses on the natural history of untreated stroke and impact of antiplatelet drugs on that situation. The natural history of TIA and completed stroke shows that risk of subsequent stroke (fatal or nonfatal) is greatest in the first follow-up year (about 12%), and that it decreases significantly (about 5% per year) in subsequent years to stroke rates that are a few percentage points above rates for individuals of the same age in the general population.[14] In TASS, stroke rates in aspirin-treated patients were close to 6% in year 1 (or about half the natural history rate) and increased by about 3% in each succeeding year on therapy (2% below the estimated natural history rate of 5% per year). The stroke rate in ticlopidine-treated patients was about 3% in year 1 and it also increased by about 3% in subsequent years.

These data suggest that antiplatelet drugs can reduce stroke rates after the first year from 5% to 3%, which is close to the natural history rate for asymptomatic individuals in the general population of similar age to the study patients. In year 1, the year of greatest risk, aspirin would appear to reduce risk of stroke to half that in untreated individuals. Ticlopidine reduced risk in year 1 to about 3%, which seems to be the lowest achievable rate for antiplatelet agents in either year 1 or subsequent treatment years. In summary, ticlopidine is superior to aspirin in year 1 and maintains its advantage over aspirin as long as therapy is continued. Ticlopidine is an effective drug for stroke prevention and is superior to aspirin.

Neutropenia is a safety concern for the drug which requires careful systemic monitoring of WBC values for the initial 3 months of therapy. The use of ticlopidine in place of aspirin should be an individual decision based on a personal assessment of the risk-benefit profile of both drugs and on one's comfort with ticlopidine's safety profile.

References

1. Hass WK, Easton JD, Adams HP, et al. A randomized trial comparing ticlopidine hydrochloride with aspirin for the prevention of stroke in high risk patients. *N Engl J Med* 1989;321:501–507.
2. Gent M, Easton JD, Hachinski VC, et al. The Canadian American ticlopidine study (CATS) in thromboembolic stroke. *Lancet* 1989;1(8649):1215–1220.
3. Data on file at Syntex Corporation.
4. Pisciotta V. Drug-induced agranulocytosis. *Drugs* 1978;**15**:132–143.
5. Statland BE. *Clinical Decision Levels for Lab Tests*. Medical Economic Company Inc., 1987.
6. Janzon L, Bergqvist D, Boberg J, et al. Prevention of myocardial infarction and stroke in patients with intermittent claudication; effects of ticlopidine. Results from STIMS, the Swedish Ticlopidine Multicentre Study. *J Intern Med* 1990;**227**:301–308.
7. Page Y, Tardy B, Zeni F, et al. Thrombotic thrombocytopenic purpura related to ticlopidine. *Lancet* 1991;**337**:774–776, 1219.
8. Shepard KV, Fishleder A, Lucas FV, et al. Thrombocytopenic purpura treated with plasma exchange or exchange transfusions. *West J Med* 1991;**154**:410–413.
9. UK-TIA Study Group: United Kingdom transient ischaemic attack (UK-TIA) aspirin trial: interim results. *Br Med J* 1988;**296**:316–320.
10. Peto R, Gray R, Collins R, et al. Randomised trial of prophylactic daily aspirin in British male doctors. *Br Med J* 1988;**296**:313–316.
11. Gurwitz JH, Avorn JA. The ambiguous relation between aging and adverse drug reactions. *Ann Intern Med* 1991;**114**:956–966.
12. The Dutch TIA Trial Study Group: A comparison of two doses of aspirin (30 mg vs. 283 mg a day) in patients after a transient ischemic attach or minor ischemic stroke. *N Engl J Med* 1991;**325**:1261–1304.
13. The Salt Collaborative Group: Swedish aspirin low-dose trial (SALT) of 75 mg aspirin as secondary prophylaxis after cerebrovascular ischaemic events. *Lancet* 1991;**338**:1345–1349.
14. Easton JD, Hart RG, Sherman DG, et al. Diagnosis and management of ischemic stroke. Part 1—Threatened stroke and its management. *Curr Probl Cardiol* 1983;**8**(5):1–75.

10
The Role of Ticlopidine in Prevention of Ischemic Stroke: A Benefit-Risk Assessment

J. DONALD EASTON

Introduction

Whenever new treatments are added to the therapeutic armamentarium, physicians are faced with assessing the overall benefits, risks, and costs of the treatment in order to make recommendations to their individual patients. Long-term warfarin for prevention of cardioembolic stroke in individuals with atrial fibrillation, and carotid endarterectomy and ticlopidine for threatened atherothrombotic stroke are two current examples.

Contemporary treatments for prevention of atherothrombotic stroke will be examined here briefly. The emphasis will be a review of data underpinning commonly used therapies and a discussion of benefits and risks (and expense) of various options.

The most commonly considered treatments for preventing stroke in patients with threatened atherothrombotic stroke, i.e., those who have suffered a transient or permanent retinal or cerebral ischemic event, are:

A) Treatment of atherosclerosis risk factors
B) Surgery
  Carotid endarterectomy
  Extracranial-to-intracranial bypass
C) Anticoagulation
D) Antiplatelet agents
  Aspirin
  Dipyridamole
  Ticlopidine

A brief review of the natural history of patients with threatened atherothrombotic stroke will provide a basis for understanding the relative benefits and risks of various treatments.

Atherosclerosis is a progressive disease causing increasing stenosis of arteries, often resulting in thromboembolism. Common consequences of this process are ischemic stroke, myocardial infarction, and vascular death. A recent analysis[1] reviewed data from published cerebrovascular studies to determine if it is possible

TABLE 10.1. Aggregate estimates of annual vascular event rates for individuals with various clincial manifestations of atherothrombotic cerebral vascular disease.

Clinical features	Annual probability (%)		
	Stroke[1]	Vascular death	All death
General elderly population	0.6	1.0	
Asymptomatic	1.3 (1.0–1.6)	3.4 (2.9–4.0)	5.4 (4.7–6.0)
Transient monocular blindness	2.2 (1.3–3.0)	3.5 (2.4–4.7)	4.3 (3.1–5.5)
Transient ischemic attack	3.7 (3.1–4.3)	2.3 (1.8–2.9)	4.0 (3.4–4.6)
Minor stroke	6.1 (5.7–6.6)	3.2 (2.8–3.6)	4.9 (4.3–5.4)
Major stroke	9.0 (8.0–9.9)	3.5 (2.8–4.2)	7.6 (6.7–8.5)

[1] 95% confidence interval

to predict, based on *clinical manifestations* of cerebrovascular atherosclerosis (e.g., cervical bruit, transient ischemic attack, stroke), the annual probability of having a stroke. Overview analysis revealed that risk profiles, based on clinical characteristics, can be generated and concluded that annual stroke rates are 1.3% for asymptomatic carotid stenosis; 2.2% for transient monocular blindness; 3.7% for transient ischemic attack; 6.1% for minor stroke; and 9.0% for major stroke (Table 10.1). Analysis showed that internal carotid artery occlusion also is a serious affair. Patients with TIA or minor stroke who have an internal carotid artery occlusion have a 6–7% risk for stroke annually. If their ischemic symptoms continue after identification of stenosis, the risk rises to 9% (Table 10.2). Thus there appears to be a hierarchical profile of worsening *clinical manifestations*, mirroring a hierarchical progression of increasing risk of stroke. Also, these patients with threatened stroke usually have generalized atherosclerosis and a substantial chance of having a myocardial infarction or vascular death.

Stroke is a principal cause of disability and loss of individual independence, as well as a leading cause of expense to patients and the health care system. It is estimated that the overall cost of health care for stroke was $15.8 billion in direct costs for 1990 in the United States.[2]

The magnitude of the stroke problem is clear. In the past there have been few treatments of proven benefit for its prevention and treatment. Recently, several major clinical studies have been started or completed that promise to clarify the value of old but unproven treatments, and some will provide, or already have provided, valuable new treatments.

Treatments for Prevention of Ischemic Stroke

Treatment of Atherosclerosis Risk Factors

Advancing age, family history, hypertension, diabetes mellitus, smoking, and hypercholesterolemia increase chances of future stroke. It is estimated that there are presently 50 million smokers, 50 million hypercholesterolemics (serum

TABLE 10.2. Aggregate estimates of annual vascular event rates for individuals with defined anatomic severity of atherosclerotic cerebral vascular disease.

Anatomic features	Annual probability (%)		
	Stroke[1]	Vascular death	All death
Asymptomatic stenosis			
Mild	0.4 (0.01–0.7)	2.3 (0.9–3.7)	2.8 (1.2–4.4)
Moderate	0.9 (0.2–1.6)	3.4 (1.3–5.5)	4.1 (1.8–6.5)
Severe	2.3 (0.8–3.7)	9.0 (4.8–13.2)	10.7 (6.1–15.2)
Carotid occlusion	6.6 (5.9–7.4)	4.6 (3.3–6.0)	11.7 (10.4–13.1)
Asymptomatic	6.5 (5.0–8.0)		
Symptomatic	9.1 (6.6–11.7)		

[1] 95% confidence interval

cholesterol > 240 mg/dl), and 50 million hypertensives who are untreated or inadequately treated. The contribution of these atherosclerosis risk factors has become well defined as properly conducted studies have been completed in recent years.

Treating hypertension and eliminating smoking[3] reduce the probability of suffering a stroke. No studies have been conducted to show that treating hypercholesterolemia reduces stroke probability. Nevertheless, the link to atherosclerosis and myocardial infarction makes such treatment logical and prudent.

Surgery

CAROTID ENDARTERECTOMY

Predictive values of carotid stenosis severity and risk of future stroke have been studied only in small numbers of patients and in restricted subgroups. Patients with asymptomatic carotid stenoses have an overall risk of about 1.1% each year of having a cerebral infarction. In these patients, some investigators have found that risk of stroke correlates with degree of stenosis: from 0.4% annually for mild stenoses to 2.3% annually for severe (> 70–75%) stenosis (Table 10.2). Although few data are available regarding prognosis for patients with > 90% carotid stenosis, there is a suggestion that stenoses approaching occlusion generate a high risk for stroke.[4] It may even be that preocclusive asymptomatic carotid stenoses have a worse prognosis than TIA or minor stroke without this degree of stenosis.

The European Carotid Surgery Trial[5] randomized more than 2500 patients with a carotid territory, nondisabling ischemic stroke, TIA, or retinal infarct, and a stenotic lesion in the ipsilateral carotid artery. For patients with only "mild" (0–29%) stenosis there was little 3-year risk of ipsilateral ischemic stroke, even in the absence of surgery. Thus, any 3-year benefits of surgery were small and were outweighed by its early post-operative risks. For patients with "severe" (70–99%) stenosis, however, risks of surgery were significantly outweighed by later benefits—although 7.5% had a stroke (or died) within 30 days of surgery, during the next 3 years the risks of ipsilateral ischemic stroke were an extra 2.8% for surgery-allocated patients and 16.8% for control patients (a sixfold reduction).

The North American Symptomatic Carotid Endarterectomy Trial (NASCET)[3] entered patients with transient cerebral or retinal ischemia or minor stroke in the arterial territory distal to a 30–99% carotid stenosis. NASCET stopped early for patients with a > 70% stenosis because of a positive result. During the first 18 months of follow-up, 24% of these patients with severe stenosis in the medical group experienced a stroke on the ipsilateral side. The rate for *all ipsilateral stroke* at 2 years was 26%, for a calculated average annual event rate of 15.1%.

These two studies provide the first robust prospectively collected data on the outcome of symptomatic patients with angiographically documented, high-grade carotid stenoses. The stroke rate was very high in unoperated patients in spite of the fact that they were taking aspirin. It is clear that a recent TIA or minor stroke, plus high-grade carotid stenosis, identifies a group of patients at very high risk for stroke within 18 months.

If *asymptomatic* individuals with severe carotid stenoses turn out to have a particularly high risk of stroke, and if the several studies of carotid endarterectomy for asymptomatic stenosis that are in progress show a benefit for the operation, the issue of identifying high-grade stenoses in asymptomatic patients may become an important one. Assessment of the overall role, timing, and value of carotid endarterectomy will be some years in evaluation.

EXTRACRANIAL-TO-INTRACRANIAL BYPASS

A large, multicenter study[6] was conducted to determine the value of extracranial-to-intracranial bypass surgery in the prevention of stroke in patients with major athero-occlusive disease. Surgery was shown to be of no value, and this operation has been largely abandoned for this indication.

Warfarin Anticoagulation

Anticoagulation is not commonly used for prevention of atherothrombotic stroke. In the United States there have been only a few randomized studies in patients with threatened stroke, all done in the 1960s.[7] The total number of randomized patients studied was 178 with TIA, 304 with progressing stroke, and 895 with completed stroke. None of these studies meet modern standards of clinical trial methodology. Consequently, we cannot presently conclude anything definitive about the efficacy of anticoagulation in prevention of atherothrombotic stroke. We should take the view that anticoagulation has not been shown to be either valuable or valueless.

There has been renewed interest in anticoagulation because of several studies published in recent years. One of these, the Oslo Myocardial Infarction Trial,[8] was a study involving 1200 patients in Norway who had suffered myocardial infarction and were randomized to either anticoagulation or placebo therapy. Although investigators were studying primarily the anticoagulation effect on myocardial infarction and vascular death, they found a 55% risk reduction for stroke. Petersen et al.[9] reported, based on a small placebo-controlled clinical trial, a benefit for low-level anticoagulation in preventing strokes in patients with nonrheumatic atrial fibrillation. Patients were randomized to either aspirin, warfarin, or placebo to determine effect on stroke outcome. Shortly thereafter, in the United States, the Stroke Prevention in Atrial Fibrillation Study Group (SPAF) published a preliminary report of their trial.[10] The study involved patients with nonrheumatic atrial fibrillation randomized to treatment with either warfarin (prothrombin time 1.3 to 1.8 times control), aspirin (325 mg daily), or placebo. After 17 months, it was decided to stop the trial's placebo arm because treatment with both aspirin and warfarin was significantly better than placebo. The trial is continuing to compare relative efficacy of warfarin and aspirin.

More recently, the Boston Area Anticoagulation Trial for Atrial Fibrillation Investigators[11] reported on results of their unblinded randomized trial to determine effect of low-dose warfarin on stroke risk in patients with nonrheumatic atrial fibrillation. There was an 86% risk reduction in stroke for warfarin over control. The death rate was 2.3% yearly in the warfarin group and 6% in the control group, and the major hemorrhage rate was very low and equal in the two groups.

Finally, the Canadian Atrial Fibrillation Anticoagulation Study,[12] a randomized double-blind, placebo-controlled trial, recently stopped early because of the positive trial results described above. The target range of anticoagulation was an international normalized ratio of 2.0 to 3.0. Risk reduction in the warfarin group was 37% for the primary outcome cluster of nonlacunar stroke, nonbrain embolism, and fatal or intracranial hemorrhage. Fatal or major bleeding occurred at annual rates of 2.5% on warfarin and 0.5% on placebo.

Because many strokes in patients with atrial fibrillation are likely to be atherothrombotic rather than cardioembolic, the anticoagulation trials noted above suggest it is worth another careful look at warfarin's efficacy in prevention of noncardiogenic atherothrombotic stroke, especially since many physicians are now using low-level anticoagulation, and bleeding complications are fewer than they were in earlier studies. A large multicenter study is about to begin which will compare aspirin to warfarin for prevention of cerebral infarction in patients who have had a previous atherothrombotic stroke.

Antiplatelet Agents

Results of the many clinical trials assessing the value of aspirin, dipyridamole, and ticlopidine have been reviewed in detail in earlier chapters. A personal summary assessment of their *relative values* is discussed below.

Overall Benefit-Risk for Available Therapies for Prevention of Atherothrombotic Stroke

This assessment will consider the following three issues: 1) risks of ischemic cerebrovascular disease; 2) benefits of each treatment in reducing risk; and 3) risks of each treatment therapy.

Risks of Ischemic Cerebrovascular Disease

The "risk" of stroke has been discussed. It is a spectrum, from relatively low risk in healthy, middle-aged individuals with no atherosclerosis risk factors to high risk in patients who have survived a completed stroke. Stroke consequences have been considered briefly in terms of loss of life, loss of independence and need for hospitalization, rehabilitation, long-term nursing care, etc. Annual financial costs of stroke are estimated at $15.8 billion in direct costs in the United States alone.

Benefits of Each Treatment in Reducing Risk

TREATMENT OF ATHEROSCLEROTIC RISK FACTORS

Treatment of atherosclerotic risk factors has proven to be beneficial. If individuals could lose weight, lower their blood pressure, lower their blood cholesterol, and stop smoking, at no financial or emotional cost, this treatment would be embraced by everyone. The fact that there are 50 million smokers, 50 million hypercholesterolemics, and 50 million inadequately treated hypertensives in the United States suggests the situation is not a simple one.

SURGERY

The benefits of carotid endarterectomy in patients who have experienced TIA or minor stroke have been discussed. It is a valuable operation for symptomatic patients with stenoses greater than 70% and who are considered reasonable risks for surgery, at least if their symptoms are of recent onset. There is no apparent place for extracranial-intracranial arterial bypass surgery in these patients.

ANTICOAGULATION

There is no currently defined place for long-term anticoagulation in preventing or treating atherothrombotic stroke; even though anticoagulants are used for this purpose, their value is unproven.

Aspirin

Plain aspirin is inexpensive and effective. It reduces vascular outcomes in patients with atherosclerosis—relative risk reduction is about 30% for stroke and myocardial infarction, 22% for stroke and death, and 15% for vascular mortality. It is probable that moderate and high-dose aspirin are similar in efficacy for stroke prevention,[13] but this has not been proven. Low-dose aspirin, such as 75 mg a day or less, appears to prevent stroke as well as moderate doses.[13,14] Side-effects of high-dose aspirin are more frequent than with low doses.

Sulfinpyrazone and Dipyridamole

Four cerebrovascular randomized trials evaluating sulfinpyrazone vs. placebo and three trials evaluating sulfinpyrazone vs. aspirin showed more events in the sulfinpyrazone than in the aspirin and placebo groups.[15]

One small trial[16] compared dipyridamole to placebo in patients with cerebrovascular disease, and there was no difference in outcomes in the two groups. No other studies have compared dipyridamole alone to placebo or aspirin. Neither has dipyridamole plus aspirin been shown to be better than aspirin alone in head-to-head comparisons.

All in all, sulfinpyrazone and dipyridamole appear to add nothing important over aspirin alone for stroke prevention.

Ticlopidine

It can be very difficult to compare the relative value of two medications, in this case ticlopidine and aspirin. Assessment will vary according to several factors:

1. Number of studies analyzed (e.g., one small, unblinded study; one large, double-blinded study; etc.).
2. Types of analyses used (e.g., intention-to-treat; efficacy (explanatory); on treatment).
3. Outcome events that are measured (e.g., all stroke; disabling stroke; fatal stroke; stroke, MI, and vascular death; stroke and all death; men only; women only; men and women, etc.).
4. Observation time of the treatment (e.g., 1 year of treatment; 3 years of treatment; etc.).

Table 10.3 shows the cumulative events per 100 patient-years and relative risk reduction for ticlopidine compared to aspirin in the Ticlopidine Aspirin Stroke Study (TASS).[17] TASS involved more than 3000 patients with TIA or minor stroke in a direct comparison of ticlopidine and aspirin to determine their effect on several cumulative outcome events over the nearly 6 years of the trial. These TASS data appear to be the best available for directly assessing benefits

TABLE 10.3 Cumulative events per 100 patient-years and relative risk reduction (RRR) for ticlopidine compared to aspirin in the TASS.

Outcome events & observation time	Intention-to-treat analysis (%)			On-treatment analysis (%)		
	Aspirin	Ticlopidine	RRR	Aspirin	Ticlopidine	RRR
Nonfatal & fatal stroke at 1 yr	6.24	3.36	46	6.41	3.36	48
Nonfatal & fatal stroke at 2 yrs	9.91	7.36	26	9.81	7.63	22
Nonfatal & fatal stroke at 3 yrs	12.72	10.01	21	13.01	10.34	21
Nonfatal & fatal stroke at 4 yrs	15.74	13.87	12	16.55	13.15	21
Nonfatal & fatal stroke at 5 yrs	18.75	16.30	13	18.07	13.75	24
Stroke & death at 1 yr	8.79	5.18	41	7.91	4.59	42
Stroke & death at 2 yrs	14.55	11.61	20	12.56	10.26	18
Stroke & death at 3yrs	19.36	17.04	12	16.64	14.46	13
Stroke & death at 3 yrs	25.23	232.23	7.9	21.78	19.85	9
Stroke & death at 3 yrs	31.38	28.42	9.4	24.89	21.90	12
Stroke, MI & vascular death at 1 yr	8.69	5.39	38	8.49	5.16	39
Stroke, MI & vascular death at 2 yrs	13.94	11.56	17	12.79	10.88	15
Stroke, MI & vascular death at 3 yrs	18.20	16.56	9	17.28	15.52	10
Stroke, MI & vascular death at 4 yrs	22.83	23.23, −2	22.67	21.41	6	
Stroke, MI & vascular death at 5 yrs	27.08	26.23	3	26.01	22.75	13

of ticlopidine vs. aspirin. In attempting to reduce data in the table to a few useful and meaningful numbers, it is necessary to make certain selections and judgments. The reader can choose according to his or her preference. Personal choices and a therapeutic rationale will be described.

First, *disabling and fatal stroke* and *stroke, MI*, and *vascular death* are the most important outcomes to assess. In TASS, *disabling stroke* was not distinguished and recorded, so it is necessary to use *nonfatal and fatal stroke*.

Second, of special interest is the effect of medications on patients who have the disease of interest (not those with some other disease who were inadvertently randomized) *and* are actually taking the medication. The on-treatment analyses are good measures of this actual treatment effect, so a good case can be made for using them. However, intention-to-treat analyses are crucial in assessing the trial's overall validity in the real life situation, thus intention-to-treat analyses are preferred (see Chapter 2).

Third, the optimal observation time of the treatment is 1 or 2 years, because it is not possible to sustain a 40–50% risk reduction beyond 2 years. There are good data, albeit from several years ago, indicating that the overall expected stroke rates in the elderly, predominantly male population, including those symptomatic for cerebral vascular disease, is about 1–2% yearly.[1,18] In the TASS intention-to-treat analysis, the cumulative stroke rate on aspirin from year 1 to year 2 was only 3.7% (Table 10.4). Thus, a further 50% reduction from ticlopidine would reduce the rate to the 1–2% one expects for the general elderly population. The cumulative stroke rate on aspirin from year 2 to year 3 was only 2.8%, so

TABLE 10.4. Cumulative strokes per 100 patient-years by intention-to-treat analysis.

	Treatment		
	Natural history[1] (%)	Aspirin (%)	Ticlopidine (%)
Stroke at 1 year	12	6.24 (48)[2]	3.36 (72)
Stroke at 2 years	20	9.91 (50)	7.36 (63)
Stroke at 3 years	25	12.72 (49)	10.01 (60)
Stroke at 4 years	30	15.74 (48)	13.87 (54)
Stroke at 5 years	35	18.75 (46)	16.30 (53)

[1] Derived from Reference number 19.
[2] Numbers in ( ) indicate the relative risk reduction compared to placebo.

a further 50% reduction would take it to 1.4%. This is virtually impossible given TASS's older population with cerebrovascular disease.

Ticlopidine data show a similar pattern to aspirin. In year 1, ticlopidine reduced risk of stroke by nearly 50% over aspirin (from 6.24% on aspirin to 3.36% on ticlopidine). Thereafter, stroke rate in the ticlopidine group increased by about 3% per year, the same increase as on aspirin.

Because there was no placebo group in the TASS trial, perhaps it is instructive to compare the aspirin and ticlopidine results with the natural history for TIAs derived from an overview analysis of published data (Table 10.4). Natural history data suggest that patients with TIA have a cumulative stroke probability of about 12% in 1 year; 20% by 2 years; 25% by 3 years; 30% by 4 years; and 35% by 5 years.[19] These data indicate that the highest risk period for stroke is the first 1 to 2 years after onset of TIAs, and thereafter, stroke rate is approximately 5% per year. Table 10.6 shows how the TASS data compare to these historical natural history data, and placebo event rates in other similar trials. It can be estimated that overall risk reduction for ticlopidine relative to placebo is approximately 60% for stroke.

From this analysis it is clear that the natural rate for stroke is high early after onset of TIA and it declines thereafter. Aspirin reduces stroke rate by about 50% in the first year, but its risk reduction declines thereafter. Similarly, ticlopidine reduces risk by about 50% over aspirin in the first year (72% over the natural rate), and its risk reduction similarly declines thereafter.

Relative risk reduction declines with each year, even though the difference in events between the two treatments (which is 3%) is sustained—this is a ratio issue. In the first year 3% less strokes (6% ASA and 3% ticlopidine) represent a 50% reduction, whereas in subsequent years, the ratio decreases even while the 3% differential is maintained. By year 5, the aspirin rate is 18%, and ticlopidine is 15%, so relative risk reduction is only 20% (18–15 18 = 20).

In summary, in assessing ticlopidine's value compared to aspirin for prevention of stroke in patients with TIA and minor stroke, it is preferable to use the following: the data from TASS; outcomes of nonfatal and fatal stroke, plus stroke, MI, and vascular death; intention-to-treat analyses; and observation time

TABLE 10.5. Author's intention-to-treat analysis and interpretation of the TASS[1] data.

Outcome events and observatoni time	Aspirin (%)	Ticlopidine (%)	RRR[2] (%)
Nonfatal and fatal stroke at 1 year	6.24	3.36	46
Nonfatal and fatal stroke at 2 years	9.91	7.36	26
Stroke, MI and vascular death at 1 year	8.69	5.39	38
Stroke, MI and vascular death at 2 years	13.94	11.56	17

[1] Ticlopidine American Stroke Study.
[2] Relative risk reduction.

of the treatment of 1 or 2 years. These results are shown in Table 10.5. Clearly, ticlopidine is more effective than aspirin for preventing stroke in these patients. Several other trials also have demonstrated the benefit of ticlopidine in stroke prevention (see Chapters 6, 7 and 8).

The Canadian American Stroke Study (CATS)[20] is the only trial limited to survivors of a major stroke in which treatment has been demonstrated to significantly reduce incidence of stroke recurrence. Only two other trials have investigated the use of antiplatelet agents for stroke prevention in patients with *major* strokes only and both were negative.[21,22] The overall risk reductions obtained in CATS, using the Cox model and an efficacy analysis, were: fatal or nonfatal stroke—34%; stroke, MI, or vascular death—30%.

RISKS, COSTS, AND MONITORING STRINGENCY OF EACH THERAPY

The final consideration in this benefit-risk analysis is treatment risk, which must be balanced against the substantial hazards of cerebrovascular disease. All forms of treatment have a variety of risk, ranging from minor discomfort to life-threatening events. In view of the seriousness of *disease risks* faced by patients with cerebrovascular disease, it is proposed to only consider *treatment risks* of like seriousness. Thus, minor inconveniences and discomforts of a given therapy will not be given the same weight as potentially life-threatening consequences of therapy.

Atherosclerosis Risk Factors

Treatment of atherosclerotic risk factors has proven to be beneficial. Some individuals will not or cannot adhere to the treatment regimen. Additionally, the newer antihypertensive and antilipid medications can be very expensive. Many patients taking them are elderly, on low incomes and on several additional expensive drugs. The main "risk" of reducing atherosclerosis risk factors can be financial ruin for the patient!

Surgery

There are several downsides to carotid endarterectomy. Presently, patients being considered for surgery must submit to the potential risk and expense of vascular studies. They then have the risk and expense of surgery. Carotid endarterectomy often has a major morbidity and mortality rate of 6–8%.[23,24] In the North American Symptomatic Carotid Endarterectomy Trial, the stroke and death rate attributable to the operation in the 30 days postrandomization, however, was only 2.2% (5.5% in the surgery group − 3.3% in the medical group = 2.2% "excess surgical morbidity and mortality") and was 1.1% for *major stroke and death*. Obviously, the high rates often reported are partially attributable to the natural event rates of the early days after onset of symptoms. Currently the average cost of the surgery in the United States is about $12,000–15,000. Carotid endarterectomy does not treat, of course, the associated generalized atherosclerosis.

Anticoagulation

In the four recent trials[9–12] testing warfarin for prevention of stroke in patients with nonrheumatic atrial fibrillation, the rate of serious hemorrhage averaged 1.2% yearly in patients randomized to warfarin. The average target international normalized ratio for the prothrombin times was 2.7. Additionally, these patients required regular testing and management of their prothrombin times.

While the expense, nuisance for the patient and physician, and serious hemorrhage rate are substantial, patients with nonrheumatic atrial fibrillation have a five to six times higher likelihood of experiencing a stroke each year than their age-matched counterparts without atrial fibrillation. This is a stroke risk of the same magnitude as new onset TIA. Most physicians conclude that benefits outweigh risks and are anticoagulating these patients, even though the Stroke Prevention in Atrial Fibrillation study[10] showed that aspirin also reduced stroke risk. It will be interesting to see what physicians will do if the Stroke Prevention in Atrial Fibrillation II study shows that warfarin reduces the risk of stroke by only a modest amount more than aspirin. How much benefit from warfarin will be required to outweigh the expense, nuisance, and 1.2% serious hemorrhage rate?

Antiplatelet Agents

Aspirin. The main risks associated with aspirin are gastrointestinal upset, and gastric erosion or ulceration with bleeding. In trials using 1000–1300 mg daily, the incidence of serious gastrointestinal hemorrhage requiring hospitalization was about 2.5% over the 2–4 year observation period.[17,25] The TASS trial observed a 2.4% incidence of trial terminations due to hemorrhagic complications of aspirin. When 300 mg or less are used, the serious hemorrhage incidence is 1.0–1.5%, perhaps lower.

Dipyridamole. Dipyridamole is moderately expensive and has not been shown to be better than aspirin alone.

Ticlopidine. Ticlopidine's two major downside issues are expense and the serious adverse reactions that occur in a little less than 1–2% of patients. Otherwise, ticlopidine-related side effects are relatively minor. Cost varies from

TABLE 10.6. Patients on Ticlopidine with serious adverse events in TASS[1]and CATS.[2]

Severe adverse event	CATS	TASS
Neutropenia (severe, neutrophils < 450/cu mm)	4	13
Hemorrhage (severe or primary termination reason)	5	5
Hepatic reactions (severe)	1	2
Total	10	20
% of patients	1.89%	1.32%
Total patientes at risk	530	1518

[1] TASS—Ticlopidine AspirinStroke Study
[2] CATS—Canadian American Stroke Study

country to country but is similar to costs of the newer antihypertensive and antilipid drugs.

Ticlopidine can cause several mild to moderate adverse reactions, but the serious adverse reactions are limited to neutropenia, hemorrhagic events and hepatic reactions. Table 10.6 summarizes the number of serious adverse events in TASS and CATS. The overall rate of these serious adverse reactions was 1.3–1.9%, which is similar to the rate of serious hemorrhagic complications with aspirin and warfarin. An additional 4% of patients will be unable to take ticlopidine because of skin rash or diarrhea.

The risk of neutropenia requires patients to have six white blood cell counts, at 2-week intervals, from initiation of treatment. Unlike anticoagulation treatment, long-term monitoring is not required.

An Assessment of the Benefit-to-Risk Ratio of Ticlopidine

Ticlopidine and aspirin are the two antiplatelet agents of primary interest in comparing benefit-risk profiles. Consequently, ticlopidine's benefit-risk in patients with threatened stroke requires comparison to "no therapy" and the standard drug, aspirin.

It is reasonable, in constructing a benefit-risk profile, to compare serious risks of treatment to serious risks of no treatment. Serious risks of no treatment in this case are death or disability. Equivalent serious risks for aspirin should be severe allergic reactions; life-threatening gastrointestinal bleeding; ulceration requiring hospitalization, transfusions or surgery; and intracranial bleeding or death.

The benefits of no therapy are avoidance of angiographic and surgical complications, lack of drug intolerance or toxicity, and lack of expense for procedures and medications.

In assessing the benefit for aspirin over placebo, results have varied from study to study, from men to women, from intention-to-treat to on-treatment analyses, and from the early months to the late months of the various studies. Nonetheless, some aggregate numbers emerge from an overview of the large number of studies that have been conducted. The benefit of aspirin, in reducing the hard outcome of *stroke plus death*, is about a 22% reduction of these events. Risks are a 0.5–1.0% yearly incidence of serious gastrointestinal complications, depending on aspirin dose. The expense of the medication is low. One can conclude from these data that therapeutic gains on mortality and morbidity for aspirin over placebo more than offset risks for hemorrhagic complications on aspirin compared to placebo, whether one measures "any GI bleed" or "serious GI bleed."

As in the assessment of aspirin's benefits, a number of factors determine the aggregate benefit one attributes to ticlopidine. Ticlopidine's benefit over aspirin on reducing *nonfatal and fatal stroke* is 46% at 1 year, and 26% at 2 years (Table 10.4). The benefit on reducing *stroke, MI, and vascular death* at 1 year is 38% and at 2 years is 17%. Total incidence of serious or potentially life-threatening problems for ticlopidine is about 1.6%, which is the *yearly* rate of serious hemorrhagic complications with warfarin. Ticlopidine's cost is substantially more than aspirin's. However, this cost does not take into consideration the substantial savings of medical care expense for strokes that are prevented.

From these data one can conclude that the therapeutic superiority of ticlopidine over aspirin is maintained even when the slightly higher morbidity attributable to ticlopidine, plus its expense and nuisance of monitoring for the first 6 weeks of treatment, are added to the equation. A great deal of the final judgment on relative value rests on the value assigned to prevented strokes and vascular deaths.

Conclusions

Stroke often causes death or major disability with loss of independence. Patients with cerebrovascular disease are at great risk for serious or fatal vascular events, and about one-third of patients not on antithrombotic treatment will suffer a stroke, MI, or death during the 3 to 5 years following the initial cerebrovascular incident. Financial costs of stroke are enormous, and preventive therapy is the primary defense.

Carotid endarterectomy is widely used to reduce risk of stroke in patients with TIA and minor stroke. While the operation's risks and expense are substantial, benefits are dramatic if the surgery is performed with a low complication rate. Weighing these several factors leads most physicians in North America to recommend carotid endarterectomy *in properly selected patients*. Following surgery, patients should be on medical treatment, as the risk of further vascular events is substantial.

Anticoagulants are used for the prevention of cerebral ischemia in a variety of settings. Warfarin is clearly beneficial for long-term prevention of stroke in patients with atrial fibrillation and some prosthetic heart valves in spite of the risk of hemorrhagic complications. Its efficacy for prevention of atherothrombotic stroke remains controversial. The lack of proven benefit, coupled with the risk of hemorrhages, cost of monitoring, and nuisance of management, limit its use for this indication.

A number of well-designed multicenter clinical trials have established the benefit of aspirin for preventing stroke in patients with TIA and minor stroke. The overall risk reduction is about 30% for nonfatal stroke, 22% for stroke and death, and 15% for death. Other antiplatelet drugs, such as dipyridamole and sulfinpyrazone, have not been demonstrated to be better than aspirin alone.

Several trials have demonstrated ticlopidine's benefit in stroke prevention in women and men, and in patients with major strokes as well as those with TIA and minor strokes. The TASS trial demonstrated that the benefits of ticlopidine over aspirin on reducing nonfatal and fatal stroke are 46% at 1 year and 26% at 2 years (Table 10.4). The benefits of ticlopidine over aspirin on reducing stroke, MI, and vascular death at 1 year are 38% and at 2 years are 17%. The CATS trial demonstrated that ticlopidine is effective in patients with major stroke, and the overall risk reduction over placebo was 34% for fatal or nonfatal stroke and 30% for stroke, MI, or vascular death. Risk of treatment with ticlopidine, in terms of major adverse effects, is comparable to that of aspirin therapy, while ticlopidine requires careful monitoring of the white blood cell count for the first 3 months on treatment.

Primary prevention is also an important therapeutic objective, as many patients with stroke (83% in the CATS trial) have no warning TIA. This issue has not been adequately studied.

References

1. Wilterdink JL, Easton JD. Outcome rates for vascular events in patients with atherosclerotic cerebral vascular disease. *Arch Neurol* 1992;**49**:857–863.
2. American Heart Association, *1991 Heart and Stroke Facts*, 1991; p. 13.
3. North American Symptomatic Carotid Endarterectomy Trial Collaborators. Beneficial effect of carotid endarterectomy in symptomatic patients with high-grade carotid stenosis. *N Engl J Med* 1991;**325**:445–453.
4. Shinton R, Beevers G. Meta-analysis of relation between cigarette smoking and stroke. *Br Med J* 1989;**298**:789–794.
5. European Carotid Surgery Trialists' Collaborative Group. MRC European Carotid Surgery Trial: interim results for symptomatic patients with severe (70–99%) or with mild (0–29%) carotid stenosis. *Lancet* 1991;**337**:1235–1243.
6. The EC/IC Bypass Study Group: Failure of extracranial-intracranial arterial bypass to reduce the risk of ischemic stroke: results of an international randomized trial. *N Engl J Med* 1985;**313**:1191–1200.
7. Easton JD, Hart RG, Sherman DG, Kaste M. Diagnosis and management of ischemic stroke. Part I. Threatened stroke and its management. *Curr Probl Cardiol* 1983;**8**:1–76.
8. Smith P, Arnesen H, Holme I. The effect of warfarin on mortality and reinfarction after myocardial infarction. *N Engl J Med* 1990;**323**:147–152.
9. Petersen P, Godtfredsen J, Boysen G, Andersen ED, Andersen B. Placebo-controlled, randomized trial of warfarin and aspirin for prevention of thromboembolic complications in chronic atrial fibrillation: the Copenhagen AFASAK Study. *Lancet* 1989;**1**: 175–178.

10. Stroke Prevention in Atrial Fibrillation Investigators. Stroke prevention in atrial fibril-lation study: final results. *Circulation* 1991;**84**:527–539.
11. The Boston Area Anticoagulation Trial for Atrial Fibrillation Investigators. The effect of low-dose warfarin on the risk of stroke in patients with nonrheumatic atrial fibrilla-tion. *N Engl J Med* 1990;**323**:1505–1511.
12. Connolly SJ, Laupacis A, Gent M, Roberts RS, Cairns JA, Joyner C. Canadian atrial fibrillation anticoagulation (CAFA) study. *JACC* 1991;**18**:349–355.
13. Dyken ML, Barnett HJM, Easton JD, Fields, WS, Fuster V, Hachinski VC, Norris JW, Sherman DG. *Stroke* 1992;**23**:(in press October).
14. The Dutch TIA Trial Study Group. A comparison of two doses of aspirin (30 mg vs. 283 mg a day) in patients after a transient ischemic attack or minor ischemic stroke. *N Engl J Med* 1991;**325**:1261–1266.
15. Antiplatelet Trialists' Collaboration: Secondary prevention of vascular disease by prolonged antiplatelet treatment. *Br Med J* 1988;**296**:320–331.
16. Acheson J, Danta G, Hutchinson EC. Controlled trial of dipyridamole in cerebral vascular disease. *Br Med J* 1969;**1**:614–615.
17. Hass WK, Easton JD, Adams HP Jr, Pryse-Phillips W, Molony BA, Anderson S, Kamm B. A randomized trial comparing ticlopidine hydrochloride with aspirin for the preven-tion of stroke in high-risk patients. *N Engl J Med* 1989;**321**:501–507.
18. Wolf PA. An overview of the epidemiology of stroke. *Stroke* 1990;**21**(supp II)4–6.
19. Easton JD, Hart RG, Kaste M, Sherman DG. Diagnosis and management of ischemic stroke. Part I. Threatened stroke and its management. *Curr Probl Cardiol* 1983;**8**:1–76.
20. Gent M, Blakely JA, Easton JD, Ellis DJ, Hachinski VC, Harbison JW, et al. The Canadian American ticlopidine study (CATS) in thromboembolic stroke. *Lancet* 1989;**1**:1215–1220.
21. Gent M, Blakely JA, Hachinski VC, et al. A secondary prevention, randomized trial of suloctidil in patients with a recent history of thromboembolic stroke. *Stroke* 1985;**16**:416–424.
22. Swedish Cooperative Study. High-dose acetylsalicylic acid after cerebral infarction. *Stroke* 1987;**18**:325–334.
23. Brott TG, Labutta RJ, Kempezinski RF. Changing patterns in the practice of carotid endarterectomy in a large metropolitan area. *JAMA* 1986;**225**:2609–2612.
24. Fode NC, Sundt TM Jr, Robertson JT, Peerless SJ, Shields CB. Multicenter retrospective review of results and complications of carotid endarterectomy in 1981. *Stroke* 1986;**17**:370–376.
25. UK-TIA Study Group. United Kingdom transient ischaemic attack (UK-TIA) aspirin trial: final results. *J Neurol Neurosurg Psychiat* 1991;**54**:1044–1054.

Index